Diseases of the Ear, Nose and Throat

MB, B................

Consultant Otolaryngologist
Royal Hallamshire Hospital
and Sheffield Children's Hospital
Sheffield

Honorary Senior Clinical Lecturer
in Otolaryngology
University of Sheffield

Ninth Edition

Blackwell
Science

© 2002 by Blackwell Science Ltd
a Blackwell Publishing Company
Editorial Offices:
Osney Mead, Oxford OX2 0EL, UK
  Tel: +44 (0)1865 206206
Blackwell Science Inc., 350 Main Street, Malden, MA 02148-5018, USA
  Tel: +1 781 388 8250
Blackwell Science Asia Pty, 54 University Street, Carlton, Victoria 3053, Australia
  Tel: +61 (0)3 9347 0300
Blackwell Wissenschafts Verlag, Kurfürstendamm 57, 10707 Berlin, Germany
  Tel: +49 (0)30 32 79 060

The right of the Author to be identified as the Author of this Work has been asserted in
accordance with the Copyright, Designs and Patents Act 1988.

First published 1961
Reprinted 1962, 1965, 1967
Second edition 1968
Reprinted 1970, 1971
Third edition 1972
Reprinted 1975
Fourth edition 1976
Reprinted 1978
Fifth edition 1980
Sixth edition 1985

Reprinted 1988, 1989
Seventh edition 1991
Reprinted 1992, 1993, 1995
Four Dragons edition 1991
Reprinted 1992, 1995
Eighth edition 1996
International edition 1996
Reprinted 1999
Ninth edition 2002

Library of Congress Cataloging-in-Publication Data

Bull, P. D.
    Lecture notes on diseases of the ear, nose, and throat. — 9th ed. /
  P. D. Bull. p.   cm. — (Lecture notes on)
    Includes index.
      ISBN 0-632-06506-0 (pbk.)
      1. Otolaryngology.
      [DNLM: 1. Otorhinolaryngologic Diseases. WV 140 B935L 2002]
      I. Title: Diseases of the ear, nose, and throat. II. Title. III. Lecture notes series
        RF46 .B954 2002
        617.5'1—dc21

                                                              2001007096

ISBN 0-632-06506-0

A catalogue record for this title is available from the British Library

Set in 9/12 Gill Sans by SNP Best-set Typesetter Ltd., Hong Kong
Printed and bound in India by Replika Press PVT Ltd

For further information on Blackwell Publishing, visit our website:
www.blackwell-science.com

Contents

Preface to the Ninth Edition

This ninth edition of *Lecture Notes on Diseases of the Ear, Nose and Throat* again allows an updating of the text. We have been able to include on this occasion further colour photographs rather than line drawings which I hope will remain in the memory better and serve as reminders to the readers of the conditions that can occur within the upper aerodigestive tract. It is interesting in revising this little book every few years how much there is to change in fairly subtle ways as the specialty develops and technology improves. The trend in educational circles in the early part of the 21st century seems to be that students should learn less and less factual knowledge and there is far more concern with process and in a spirit of concordance with this (though not entire agreement), I have reduced the text of some of the chapters considerably and omitted quite a lot of details, particularly where it relates to surgical procedures. As before, I have avoided the cumbersome use of 'he or she', or 'they' as a singular pronoun and I hope that I will be forgiven again in the interest in avoiding prolixity for using 'he' to mean either gender without prejudice or favour.

Acknowledgements

I am pleased to acknowledge the invaluable help of the editorial and production departments of Blackwell Publishing who have encouraged the production of this new edition of *Lecture Notes in Diseases of the Ear, Nose and Throat*, and in particular to Fiona Goodgame and Alice Emmott.

I am grateful to my clinical colleagues for advice willingly given and for help with the illustrations. I am indebted particularly to Mark Yardley, Tim Woolford, Charles Romanowski and Tim Hodgson.

Without the skill and cooperation of the Department of Medical Illustration at the Royal Hallamshire Hospital, I would have had few images to include in this little book.

I am grateful to Alun Bull for the cover images.

P.D. Bull
January 2002

Preface to the First Edition

This book is intended for the undergraduate medical student and the house officer. It is hoped that, though elementary, it will also prove of use to the general practitioner.

Many conditions encompassed within the so-called 'specialist' subjects are commonly seen in general practice, and the practitioner is therefore obliged to be familiar with them. He is not asked to perform complex aural operations, or even to be acquainted with their details, but he is expected to appreciate the significance of headache supervening in otitis media, to treat epitaxis, and to know the indications for tonsillectomy.

Emphasis has therefore been laid on conditions that are important either because they are common or because they call for investigation or early treatment. Conversely, some are rare conditions and specialized techniques have received but scant attention, whilst others have been omitted, because the undergraduate should be protected from too much 'small print', which will clutter his mind and which belongs more properly to postgraduate studies.

The study of past examination questions should be an integral part of the preparation for any examination, and students are strongly advised to 'work-up' the examination questions at the end of the book. Time spent in this occupation will certainly not be wasted, for the questions refer, in every case, to the fundamentals of the specialty.

E.H. Miles Foxen

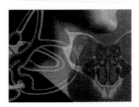

CHAPTER 1

The Ear: Some Applied Anatomy

THE PINNA

The external ear or pinna, is composed of cartilage with closely adherent perichondrium and skin. It is developed from six tubercles of the first branchial arch. Fistulae and accessory auricles result from failure of fusion of these tubercles.

THE EXTERNAL AUDITORY MEATUS

The external auditory meatus is about 25 mm in length, has a skeleton of cartilage in its outer third (where it contains hairs and ceruminous glands) and has bone in its inner two-thirds. The skin of the inner part is exceedingly thin, adherent and sensitive. At the medial end of the meatus there is the antero-inferior recess, in which wax, debris or foreign bodies may lodge.

THE TYMPANIC MEMBRANE (Fig. 1.1)

The tympanic membrane is composed of three layer — skin, fibrous tissue and mucosa. The normal appearance of the membrane is pearly and opaque, with a well-defined light reflex due to its concave shape.

THE TYMPANIC CAVITY

Medial to the tympanic membrane, the tympanic cavity is an air-containing space 15 mm high and 15 mm antero-posteriorly, although only 2 mm deep in parts. The middle ear contains the ossicular chain of malleus, incus and stapes (Fig. 1.2) and its medial wall is crowded with structures closely related to one another: the facial nerve, the round and oval windows, the lateral semicircular canal and basal turn of the cochlea. The major reason for having an air-containing middle ear is to reduce the acoustic impedance that would be caused if a sound wave in air were to be applied directly to the cochlear fluids. Without this impedance matching, 99% of the sound energy would simply be reflected at an air/fluid interface.

THE EUSTACHIAN TUBE

The Eustachian tube connects the middle-ear cleft with the nasopharynx and is responsible for the aeration of the middle ear. The tube is more

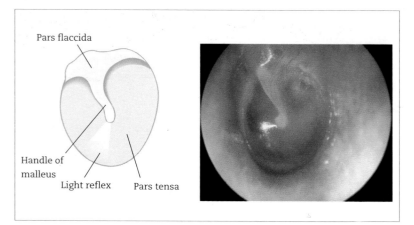

Fig. 1.1 The normal tympanic membrane (left). The shape of the incus is visible through the drum at 2 o'clock. (Courtesy of MPJ Yardley.)

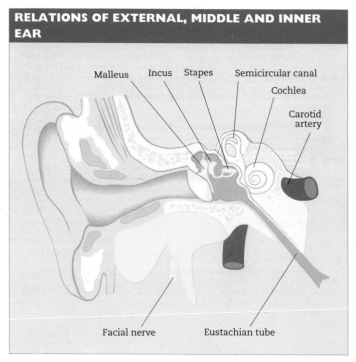

Fig. 1.2 Diagram to show the relationship between the external, middle and inner ears.

ANATOMY OF MIDDLE EAR AND MASTOID AIR CELLS

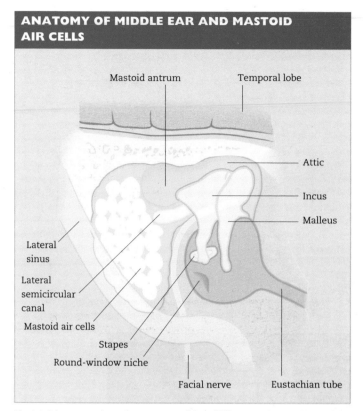

Fig. 1.3 Diagram to show the anatomy of the middle ear and mastoid air cells.

horizontal in the infant than in the adult and secretions or vomit may enter the tympanic cavity more easily in the supine position. The tube is normally closed and is opened by the palatal muscles on swallowing. This is impaired by the presence of a palatal cleft.

THE FACIAL NERVE

The facial nerve is embedded in bone in its petrous part but exits at the stylomastoid foramen (Fig. 1.3). In infants, the mastoid process is undeveloped and the nerve very superficial.

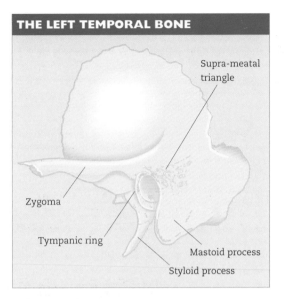

THE LEFT TEMPORAL BONE

Supra-meatal triangle

Zygoma

Tympanic ring

Mastoid process

Styloid process

Fig. 1.4 The left temporal bone.

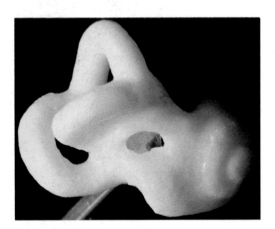

Fig. 1.5 A preparation showing the bony inner ear of semicircular canals and cochlea (Preparation by Mr S Ell.)

THE MASTOID CELLS

The mastoid cells form a honeycomb within the temporal bone, acting as a reservoir of air to limit pressure changes within the middle ear. The extent of pneumatization is very variable and is usually reduced in chronic middle-ear disease.

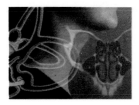

CHAPTER 2

Clinical Examination
of the Ear

The examination of the ear includes close inspection of the pinna, the external auditory canal and the tympanic membrane. Scars from any previous surgery may be inconspicuous and easily missed.

The ear is most conveniently examined with an auriscope (Fig. 2.1). Modern auriscopes have distal illumination via a fibre-optic cone giving a bright, even light. Because interpretation of the appearance depends to a

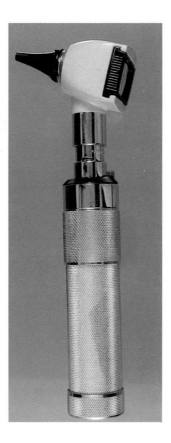

Fig. 2.1 Auriscope with halogen bulb lighting via a fibreoptic cone.

large extent on colour, it is essential that the battery should be in good condition to give a white light.

A common error in examination of the tympanic membrane is to use too small a speculum; the largest that can be inserted easily should be used. Good auriscopes are expensive but are a worthwhile investment. Important points in the examination of the ear are listed in Box 2.1.

EXAMINATION OF THE EAR

1   Look for any previous scars.
2   Examine the pinna and outer meatus by head-mirror or room lighting.
3   Remove any wax or debris by syringing, or by instruments if you are practised in this.
4   Pull the pinna gently backwards and upwards (downwards and backwards in infants) to straighten out the meatus.
5   Insert the auriscope *gently* into the meatus and see where you are going by looking *through* the instrument. If you cannot get a good view, either the speculum is the wrong size or the angulation is wrong.
6   Inspect the external canal.
7   Inspect all parts of the tympanic membrane by varying the angle of the speculum.
8   Do not be satisfied until you have seen the membrane completely.
9   The normal appearance of the membrane varies and can only be learnt by practice. Such practice will lead to the recognition of subtle abnormalities as well as the more obvious ones.

Box 2.1 Examination of the ear.

CHAPTER 3

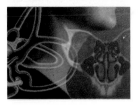

Testing the Hearing

There are three stages to testing the hearing and all are important. Audiograms can be wrong.

1   Clinical assessment of the degree of deafness.
2   Tuning fork tests.
3   Audiometry.

CLINICAL ASSESSMENT OF THE DEGREE OF DEAFNESS

By talking to the patient, the examiner quickly appreciates how well a patient can hear and this assessment continues throughout the interview. A more formal assessment is then made by asking the patient to repeat words spoken by the examiner at different intensities and distances in each ear in turn. The result is recorded as, for example, whispered voice (WV) at 150 cm in a patient with slight deafness, or conversational voice (CV) at 15 cm in a deafer individual.

If profound unilateral deafness is suspected, the good ear should be masked with a Barany noise box and the deaf ear tested by shouting into it.

The limitations of voice and whisper tests must be borne in mind; they are approximations but with practice can be a good guide to the level of hearing and will confirm the audiometric findings.

TUNING FORK TESTS

Before considering tuning fork tests it is necessary to have a basic concept of classification of deafness. Almost every form of deafness (and there are many) may be classified under one of these headings:

• conductive deafness;
• sensorineural deafness;
• mixed conductive and sensorineural deafness.

Conductive deafness (Fig. 3.1)

Conductive deafness results from mechanical attenuation of the sound waves in the outer or middle ear, preventing sound energy from reaching

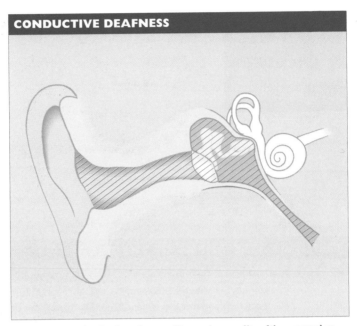

CONDUCTIVE DEAFNESS

Fig. 3.1 Conductive deafness is caused by an abnormality of the external or middle ear (shaded).

the cochlear fluids. It may be remediable by surgery and so it is important it is recognized. The hearing by bone conduction will be normal in pure conductive deafness.

Sensorineural deafness (Fig. 3.2)

Sensorineural deafness results from defective function of the cochlea or of the auditory nerve, and prevents neural impulses from being transmitted to the auditory cortex of the brain.

Mixed deafness

Mixed deafness is the term used to describe a combination of conductive and sensorineural deafness in the same ear.

RINNE'S TEST

This test compares the relative effectiveness of sound transmission through the middle ear by air conduction (AC), and bypassing the middle ear by bone conduction (BC). It is usually performed as follows: a tuning fork of 512 Hz (cycles per second) is struck and held close to the patient's ear; it is then

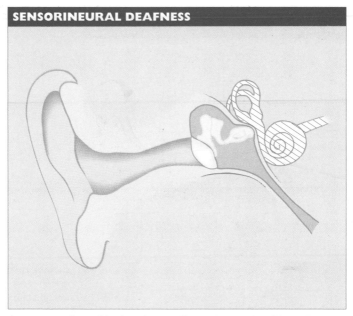

SENSORINEURAL DEAFNESS

Fig. 3.2 Sensorineural deafness is caused by an abnormality of the cochlea or the auditory nerve (shaded).

placed firmly on the mastoid process and the patient is asked to state whether it is heard better by BC or AC.

Interpretation of Rinne's test

If AC > BC – called Rinne positive – the middle and outer ears are functioning normally.

If BC > AC – called Rinne negative – there is defective function of the outer or middle ear.

Rinne's test tells you little or nothing about cochlear function. It is a test of middle-ear function.

WEBER'S TEST

This test is useful in determining the type of deafness a patient may have and in deciding which ear has the better-functioning cochlea. The base of a vibrating tuning fork is held on the vertex of the head and the patient is asked whether the sound is heard centrally or is referred to one or other ear.

In conductive deafness the sound is heard in the deafer ear.

In sensorineural deafness the sound is heard in the better-hearing ear (Figs 3.3–3.5)

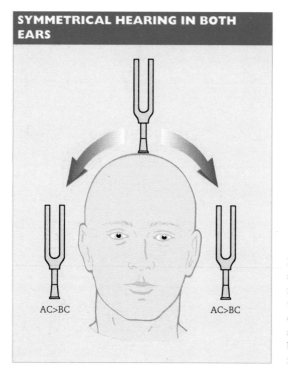

SYMMETRICAL HEARING IN BOTH EARS

AC>BC   AC>BC

Fig. 3.3 Tuning fork tests showing a positive Rinne in each ear and the Weber test referred equally to each ear, indicating symmetrical hearing in both ears with normal middle-ear function.

AUDIOMETRY

PURE TONE AUDIOMETRY

Pure tone audiometry provides a measurement of hearing levels by AC and BC and depends on the cooperation of the subject. The test should be carried out in a sound-proofed room. The audiometer is an instrument that generates pure tone signals ranging from 125 to 12000 Hz (12 kHz) at variable intensities. The signal is fed to the patient through ear phones (for AC) or a small vibrator applied to the mastoid process (for BC). Signals of increasing intensity at each frequency are fed to the patient, who indicates when the test tone can be heard. The threshold of hearing at each frequency is charted in the form of an audiogram (Figs 3.6–3.8), with hearing loss expressed in decibels (dB). Decibels are logarithmic units of relative intensity of sound energy. When testing hearing by BC, it is essential to mask the opposite ear with narrow-band noise to avoid cross-transmission of the signal to the other ear.

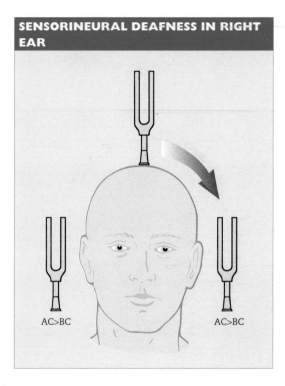

SENSORINEURAL DEAFNESS IN RIGHT EAR

AC>BC   AC>BC

Fig. 3.4 Sensorineural deafness in the right ear. The Rinne test is positive on both sides and the Weber test is referred to the left ear.

SPEECH AUDIOMETRY

Speech audiometry is employed to measure the ability of each ear to discriminate the spoken word at different intensities. A recorded word list is supplied to the patient through the audiometer at increasing loudness levels, and the score is plotted on a graph. In some disorders, the intelligibility of speech may fall off above a certain intensity level. It usually implies the presence of *loudness recruitment*—an abnormal growth of loudness perception. Above a critical threshold, sounds are suddenly perceived as having become excessively loud. This is indicative of cochlear disorder.

IMPEDANCE TYMPANOMETRY

Impedance tympanometry measures not hearing but, indirectly, the compliance of the middle-ear structures. A pure tone signal of known intensity is fed into the external auditory canal and a microphone in the ear probe measures reflected sound levels. Thus, the sound admitted to the ear can be measured. Most sound is absorbed when the compliance is maximal, and, by altering the pressure in the external canal, a measure can be made of the

CONDUCTIVE DEAFNESS IN RIGHT EAR

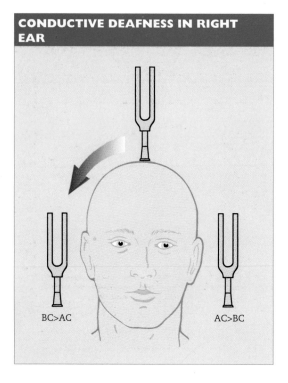

BC>AC   AC>BC

Fig. 3.5 Conductive deafness in the right ear. The Rinne test is negative on the right, positive on the left and the Weber test is referred to the right ear.

NORMAL PURE TONE AUDIOGRAM

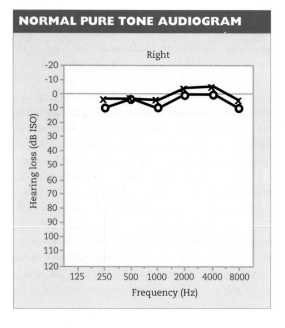

Fig. 3.6 A normal pure tone audiogram. o–o–o, right ear; x–x–x, left ear.

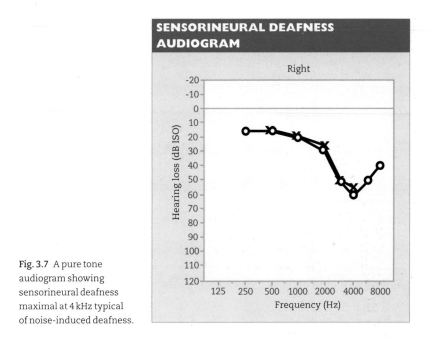

Fig. 3.7 A pure tone audiogram showing sensorineural deafness maximal at 4 kHz typical of noise-induced deafness.

compliance at different pressures. Impedance testing is widely used as a screening method for otitis media with effusion (OME) in children. If there is fluid in the middle ear, the compliance curve is flattened.

ELECTRIC RESPONSE AUDIOMETRY

Electric response audiometry is a collective term for various investigations whereby action potentials at various points within the long and complex auditory pathway can be recorded. The action potential (AP) is evoked by a sound stimulus applied to the ear either through headphones or free field, and the resulting AP is collected in a computer store. Although each AP is tiny, it occurs at the same time interval after the stimulus (usually a click of *very* short duration) and so a train of stimuli will produce an easily detectable response, while the averaging ability of the computer will average out the more random electrical activity, such as the EEG. By making the computer look at different time windows, responses at various sites in the auditory pathway can be investigated. As the response travels from the cochlea to the auditory cortex, the latency increases from about 1-4 to 300 ms.

CONDUCTIVE DEAFNESS

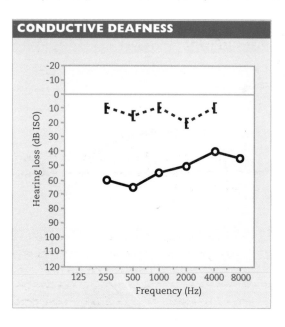

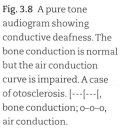

Fig. 3.8 A pure tone audiogram showing conductive deafness. The bone conduction is normal but the air conduction curve is impaired. A case of otosclerosis. [---[---[, bone conduction; o–o–o, air conduction.

There are three main responses used in clinical audiology.

1   Electrocochleogram (E Coch G), which is recorded from an electrode inserted through the ear drum onto the promontory and can be recorded under anaesthetic.

2   Brain-stem responses, recorded from external electrodes (BSER).

3   Slow vertex or cortical responses, again recorded from external electrodes (SVR or CERA).

Electric response audiometry has the unique advantage of being an objective measure of hearing requiring no cooperation from the subject. It is of value in assessing hearing thresholds in babies and small children and in cases of dispute such as litigation for industrial deafness.

Oto-acoustic emissions (OAE)

When the cochlea is subjected to a sound wave it is stimulated to produce itself an emission of sound generated within the cochlea. This can be detected and recorded and has been used as a screening test of hearing in newborn babies. It is now in routine clinical use in testing those babies who are particularly at risk of hearing problems, such as premature or hypoxic neonates, and is likely to play a part in universal screening for hearing loss.

CHAPTER 4

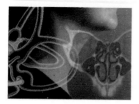

Deafness

Attention has already been drawn to the two major categories of deafness—conductive and sensorineural. The distinction is easily made by tuning fork tests, which should never be omitted.

CAUSES

There is no strict order in the list featured in Table 4.1, because the frequency with which various causes of deafness occur varies from one community to another and from one age group to another. Nevertheless, some indication is given by division into 'more common' and 'less common' groups. Always try to make a diagnosis of the cause of deafness and start by deciding whether it is conductive or sensorineural.

MANAGEMENT

The management of a number of specific conditions will be dealt with in subsequent chapters but some general comments are appropriate.

The deaf child

Early diagnosis of deafness in the infant is essential if irretrievable developmental delay is to be avoided. The health visitor should screen all babies at about 8 months of age and those failing a routine test must be referred to a specialist audiological centre without delay for more thorough investigation. Some babies are 'at risk' of deafness and are tested as soon after birth as possible. They include those affected by:

1 prematurity and low birth-weight;
2 perinatal hypoxia;
3 Rhesus disease;
4 family history of hereditary deafness;
5 intrauterine exposure to viruses such as rubella, cytomegalovirus and HIV.

The testing of babies suspected or at risk of being deaf is very specialized. The mother's assessment is very important and should always be taken seriously. She is likely to be right if she thinks her child's hearing is not normal. Testing of 'at risk' babies in the neonatal period is now carried out in many centres by the recording of otoacoustic emissions (see Chapter 3).

Conductive	Sensorineural
More common	
Wax	Presbycusis (deafness of old age)
Acute otitis media	Noise-induced (prolonged exposure to high noise level, industrial deafness, chronic otitis media disco music)
Barotrauma	Congenital (maternal rubella, cytomegalovirus, toxoplasmosis, hereditary deafness, anoxia, jaundice, congenital syphilis)
Otosclerosis	
Injury of the tympanic membrane	Drug-induced (aminoglycoside antibiotics, aspirin, quinine, some diuretics, some beta blockers)
	Menière's disease
	Late otosclerosis
	Infections (CSOM, mumps, herpes zoster, meningitis, syphilis)
Less common	
Traumatic ossicular dislocation	Acoustic neuroma
Congenital atresia of the external canal	Head injury
Agenesis of the middle ear	CNS disease (multiple sclerosis, metastases)
Tumours of the middle ear	Metabolic (diabetes, hypothyroidism, Paget's disease of bone)
	Psychogenic
	Unknown aetiology

Table 4.1 Causes of deafness.

Sudden sensorineural deafness

Sudden sensorineural deafness is an otological emergency and should be treated as seriously as would be sudden blindness. Immediate admission to hospital should be arranged, as delay may mean permanent deafness.

Sudden deafness may be unilateral or bilateral and most cases are regarded as being viral or vascular in origin. Investigation may fail to show a cause and treatment is usually with low-molecular-weight dextran, steroids and inhaled carbon dioxide. Bilateral profound deafness, especially if of sudden onset, is a devastating blow and for this reason various organizations exist to give advice and support.

Vestibular Schwannoma (Acoustic neuroma)

Vestibular Schwannoma is a benign tumour of the superior vestibular nerve in the internal auditory meatus or cerebello-pontine (CP) angle. It is usually unilateral, except in familial neurofibromatosis (NF2), when it may be bilat-

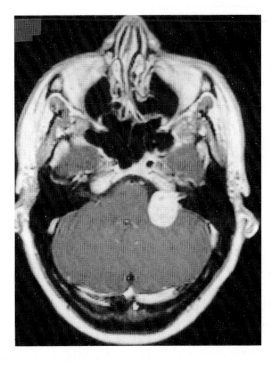

Fig. 4.1 An MR scan after gadolinium contrast showing an acoustic neuroma.

eral. In its early stages, it causes a progressive hearing loss and some imbalance. As it enlarges, it may encroach on the trigeminal nerve in the CP angle, causing loss of corneal sensation. In its advanced stage, there is raised intracranial pressure and brain stem displacement. Early diagnosis reduces the morbidity and mortality of operations. Unilateral sensorineural deafness should always be investigated to exclude a neuroma. Audiometry will confirm the hearing loss. MR scanning will identify even small tumours with certainty (Fig. 4.1).

Hearing aids

In cochlear forms of sensorineural deafness, loudness recruitment is often a marked feature. This results in an intolerance of noise above a certain threshold, and makes the provision of amplification very difficult.

The choice of hearing aids is now large. Most are worn behind the ear with a mould fitting into the meatus. If the mould does not fit well, oscillatory feedback will occur and the patient will not wear the aid. More sophisticated (and expensive) are the 'all-in-the-ear' aids, where the electronics are built into a mould made to fit the patient's ear. They give good directional hearing and, because they are individually built, the output can be matched to the patient's deafness. The current generation of hearing aids are digital, allowing more refinement in the sound processing and more control of the aid.

A recent development has been the bone-anchored hearing aid (BAHA). A titanium screw is threaded into the temporal bone and allowed to fuse to the bone (osseo-integration). A transcutaneous abutment then allows the attachment of a special hearing aid that transmits sound directly by bone conduction to the cochlea. The main application of BAHA is to patients with no ear canal, or chronic ear disease, who are unable to wear a conventional aid and is much more effective than the old-fashioned bone conductor aid.

Cochlear implants

Much research has been done, both in the USA and Europe, on the implantation of electrodes into the cochlea to stimulate the auditory nerve. The apparatus consists of a microphone, an electronic sound processor and a single or multichannel electrode implanted into the cochlea. Cochlear implantation is only appropriate for the profoundly deaf. Results, particularly with an intracochlear multichannel device, can be spectacular, with some patients able to converse easily. Most patients obtain a significant improvement in their ability to communicate and implantation has been extended for use in children. It is no longer an experimental procedure but a valuable therapeutic technique.

Lip-reading

Instruction in lip-reading is carried out much better while usable hearing persists and should always be advised to those at risk of total or profound deafness.

Electronic aids for the deaf

Amplifying telephones are easily available to the deaf and telephone companies usually provide willing advice. Many modern hearing aids are fitted with a loop inductance system to make the use of telephones easier.

Various computerized voice analysers that give a rapid visual display are also available, but these require the services of a skilled operator and are still in the developmental phase. Automatic voice recognition machines may take over this role in the foreseeable future.

CHAPTER 5

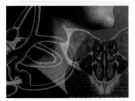

Conditions of the Pinna

Protruding ears

Sometimes unkindly known as 'bat ears', the terms protruding or prominent should be used. The underlying deformity is the absence of the antehelical fold in the auricular cartilage. Afflicted children are often teased mercilessly and surgical correction can be carried out after the age of four. Operation consists of exposing the lateral aspect of the cartilage from behind the pinna and scoring it to produce a rounded fold (Fig. 5.1).

Accessory auricles

Accessory auricles are small tags, often containing cartilage, on a line between the angle of the mouth and the tragus (Fig. 5.2). They may be multiple.

Pre-auricular sinus

Pre-auricular sinus is a small blind pit that occurs commonly anterior to the root of the helix; it is sometimes bilateral and may be familial. Recurrent infection requires excision (Fig. 5.3).

Microtia

Microtia, or failure of development of the pinna, may be associated with atresia of the ear canal (Fig. 5.2). Absence or severe malformation of the external ear, as in Treacher Collins syndrome, may be remedied by the fitting of prosthetic ears attached by bone-anchored titanium screws (see BAHA, Chapter 4, page 18). A bone-anchored hearing aid can be fitted at the same time, although it is often fitted at a much earlier age than prosthetic ears in order to allow speech development.

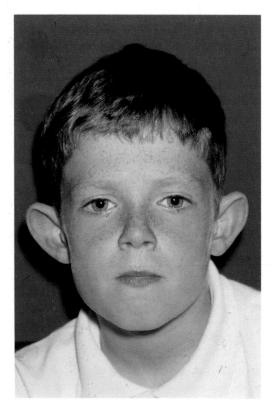

Fig. 5.1 A child with protruding ears.

TRAUMA

Haematoma

Subperichondrial haematoma of the pinna usually occurs as a result of a shearing blow (Fig. 5.4). The pinna is ballooned and the outline of the cartilage is lost. Left untreated, severe deformity will result—a cauliflower ear. Treatment consists of evacuation of the clot and the reapposition of cartilage and perichondrium by pressure dressings or vacuum drain.

AVULSION

Very rarely, avulsion of the pinna may occur. If the avulsed ear is preserved, reattachment may be possible.

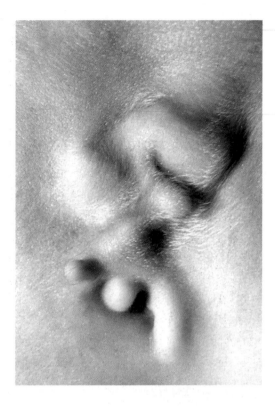

Fig. 5.2 Right ear showing congenital meatal atresia, an accessory auricle and deformity of the pinna.

INFLAMMATION

Acute dermatitis

Acute dermatitis of the pinna may occur as an extension of meatal infection in otitis externa: it is commonly caused by a sensitivity reaction to topically applied antibiotics, especially chloramphenicol or neomycin (Fig. 5.5).

TREATMENT

1   The ear canal should be adequately treated (q.v).

2   If there is any suspicion of a sensitivity reaction, topical treatment with antibiotics should be withdrawn.

3   The ear may be treated with glycerine and ichthammol, or steroid ointment may be applied *sparingly*.

4   Severe cases may require admission to hospital.

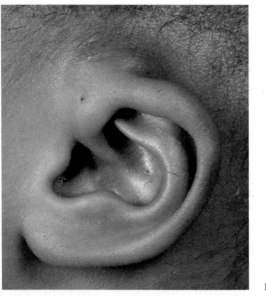

Fig. 5.3 Pre-auricular sinus.

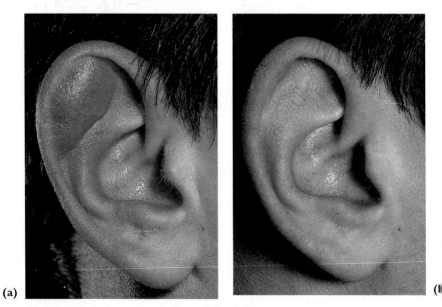

(a)   (b)

Fig. 5.4 Auricular haematoma before and after drainage.

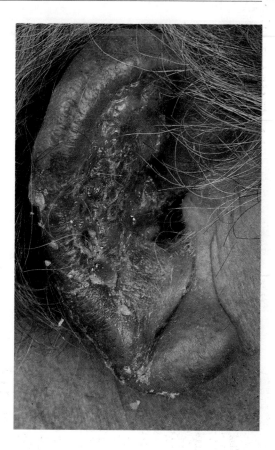

Fig. 5.5 Severe otitis externa and perichondritis of the pinna.

Dictum

If otitis externa gets worse on treatment, it is probably due to drug sensitivity. Stop the treatment.

Perichondritis

Perichondritis may follow injury to the cartilage and may be very destructive. It may follow mastoid surgery or may follow ear piercing, particularly with the modern trend for multiple perforations that may go through the cartilage. Treatment must be vigorous, with parenteral antibiotics and incision if necessary. It goes without saying that if it is due to piercing the ear, the stud should be removed.

WEDGE EXCISION

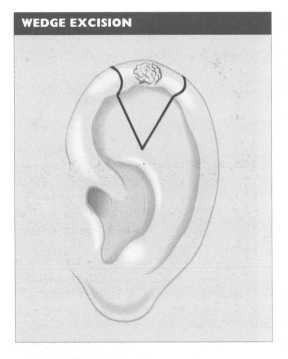

Fig. 5.6 Wedge excision of carcinoma of the pinna. The defect is repaired by direct closure.

Chondrodermatitis chronicis helicis

Chondrodermatitis chronicis helicis occurs in the elderly as a painful ulcerated lesion on the rim of the helix. It resembles a neoplasm and should be removed for histology.

TUMOURS

Squamous cell and basal cell carcinomas

These tumours occur usually on the upper edge of the pinna, and when small are easily treated by wedge excision (Fig. 5.6). Large tumours of the pinna or outer meatus will require more radical treatment, often with skin flap repair.

CHAPTER 6

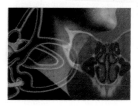

Conditions of the External Auditory Meatus

CONGENITAL

Congenital atresia (Greek: a—negative; tretos—bored through) may be of variable severity; there may be a shallow blind pit or no cavity at all. There may be associated absence of the pinna (microtia) and there may be absence or abnormality of the middle or inner ear (Fig. 5.2).

In bilateral cases the cochlear function needs to be measured carefully. If it is good, surgery may be considered. Previously an attempt would have been made to fashion an external auditory canal but better hearing results are obtained by the provision of a BAHA (see Chapter 4, page 18). At the same time any malformation of the pinna can be corrected by a prosthesis attached to a similar osseo-integrated titanium implant. Until such surgery is possible (at about age 3–4) the child with bilateral atresia of the external auditory canal will need to wear a bone conductor hearing aid held on by pressure from some sort of headband.

In unilateral cases, it is of prime importance to assess the hearing in the unaffected ear. If it is good, operation on the affected side is unnecessary. External ears can be constructed by a plastic procedure or can be replaced by prostheses anchored to the ear by adhesive or by titanium implants in the skull bone.

FOREIGN BODY

Small children often put beads, pips, paper and other objects into their own ears, but they will usually blame someone else! Adults may get a foreign body stuck in an attempt to clean the ear, e.g. with match sticks, or cotton buds.

Although the management is straightforward, several points arise.

1 Syringing is usually successful in removing a foreign body.

2 The chief danger lies in clumsy attempts to remove the foreign body and rupture of the tympanic membrane may result. Do not attempt to remove a foreign body unless you have already developed some skill with instruments.

3   If the child (or adult) is uncooperative, do not persevere but resort instead to general anaesthesia. This does not need to be done as an urgent case but can be added to a routine list.

INSECTS

Live insects, such as moths or flies, in the outer meatus produce dramatic 'tinnitus'. Peace is restored by the instillation of spirit or olive oil and the corpse can then be syringed out.

WAX

WAX IN AN EAR IS NORMAL

Wax or cerumen is produced by the ceruminous glands in the outer meatus and migrates laterally along the meatus. Some people produce large amounts of wax but many cases of impacted wax are due to the use of cotton wool buds in a misguided attempt to clean the ears.

Impacted wax may cause some deafness or irritation of the meatal skin and is most easily removed by syringing. Ear syringing is a procedure that almost any doctor or nurse is expected to carry out with skill and that the general practitioner should perform with a flawless technique. Attention must be paid to the points listed in Box 6.1.

EAR SYRINGING PROCEDURE:

1   *History.* Has the patient had a discharging ear? If any possibility of a dry perforation, do not syringe.

2   *Inspection.* If wax seems very hard, always soften over a period of one week by using warm olive oil drops nightly. In the case of exceedingly stubborn wax, the patient may be advised to use sodium bicarbonate ear drops (BPC), and there are several 'quick-acting' ceruminolytic agents on the market. Occasionally, a patient reacts badly to the use of the latter and develops otitis externa. They should certainly not be employed in the case of a patient who is known to suffer from recurrent infections of the meatal canal.

3   *Towels.* Protect the patient well with towels and waterproofs. He will not be amused by having his clothing soaked.

4   *Lighting.* Use a mirror or lamp.

5   *Solution.* Sodium bicarbonate, 4–5 g to 500 mL, or normal saline are ideal. Tapwater is satisfactory.

6   *Solution temperature.* This is vital. It should be 38°C (100°F). Any departure of more than a few degrees may precipitate the patient onto the floor with vertigo.

7   *Tools.* Metal syringes and Bacon syringes are capable of applying high pressures and the nozzle may also do damage. The preferred instrument is an electrically driven water

Continued

pump with a small hand-held nozzle and a foot operated control (Fig. 6.1). It provides an elegant means of ear syringing.

8 *Direction*. Direct stream of solution along roof of auditory canal (Fig. 6.2).

9 *Inspection*. After removal of wax, inspect thoroughly to make sure none remains. This advice might seem superfluous, but is frequently ignored.

10 *Drying*. Mop excess solution from meatal canal. Stagnation predisposes to otitis externa.

Box 6.1 Ear syringing procedure.

OTITIS EXTERNA

Otitis externa is a diffuse inflammation of the skin lining the external auditory meatus. It may be bacterial or fungal (otomycosis), and is characterized by irritation, desquamation, scanty discharge and tendency to relapse. The treatment is simple, but success is absolutely dependent upon patience, care and meticulous attention to detail.

CAUSES

Some people are particularly prone to otitis externa, often because of a narrow or tortuous external canal. Most people can allow water into their

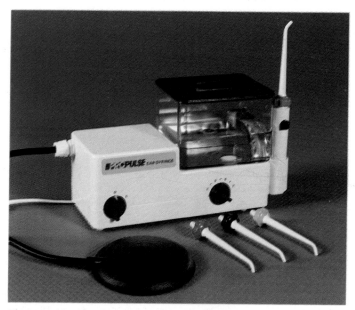

Fig. 6.1 An electric pulse pump used for ear syringing.

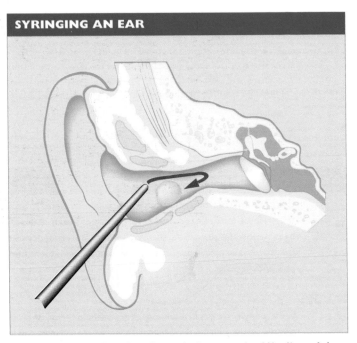

SYRINGING AN EAR

Fig. 6.2 The stream of solution when syringing an ear should be directed along the roof of the external auditory canal.

ears with impunity but in others otitis externa is the inevitable result. Swimming baths are a common source of otitis externa. Poking the ear with a finger or towel further traumatizes the skin and introduces new organisms. Further irritation occurs, leading to further interference with the ear, so causing more trauma. A vicious circle is set up.

Otitis externa may occur after staying in hotter climates than usual, where increased sweating and bathing are predisposing factors.

Underlying skin disease, such as eczema or psoriasis, may occur in the ear canal and produce very refractory otitis externa.

Ear syringing, especially if it causes trauma, may result in otitis externa.

PATHOLOGY

A mixed infection of varying organisms is not infrequent, the most commonly found types being:

- *Staphylococcus pyogenes*;
- *Pseudomonas pyocyanea*;
- diphtheroids;

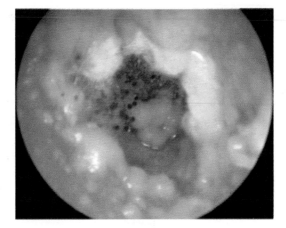

Fig. 6.3 Fungal otitis externa showing the spores of *Aspergillus niger*. (Courtesy of MPJ Yardley.)

- *Proteus vulgaris*;
- *Escherichia coli*;
- *Streptococcus faecalis*;
- *Aspergillus niger* (Fig. 6.3);
- *Candida albicans*.

SYMPTOMS

1 Irritation.
2 Discharge (scanty).
3 Pain (usually moderate, sometimes severe, increased by jaw movement).
4 Deafness.

SIGNS

1 Meatal tenderness, especially on movement of the pinna or compression of the tragus.
2 Moist debris, often smelly and keratotic, the removal of which reveals red desquamated skin and oedema of the meatal walls and often the tympanic membrane.

MANAGEMENT

Scrupulous aural toilet is the key to successful treatment of otitis externa. No medication will be effective if the ear is full of debris and pus.

Investigation

Investigation of the offending microorganism is essential. A swab should be sent for culture and it is prudent to mention the possibility of fungal infection in your request, especially if the patient has already had topical antibiotic treatment.

Aural toilet

Aural toilet must be performed and can be done most conveniently by dry mopping. Fluffed-up cotton wool about the size of a postage stamp is applied to the Jobson Horn probe and, under direct vision, the ear is cleaned with a gentle rotatory action. Once the cotton wool is soiled it is replaced. Pay particular attention to the antero-inferior recess, which may be difficult to clean. Gentle syringing is also permissible to clear the debris.

Dressings

If the otitis externa is severe, a length of 1 cm ribbon gauze, impregnated with appropriate medication, should be inserted gently into the meatus, and renewed daily until the meatus has returned to normal. If it does not do so within 7–10 days, think again!.

The following medications are of value on the dressing:

1   8% aluminium acetate;
2   10% ichthammol in glycerine;
3   ointment of gramicidin, neomycin, nystatin and triamcinolone (Tri-Adcortyl);
4   other medication may be used as dictated by the result of culture.

If *fungal otitis externa* is present, dressings of 3% amphotericin, miconazole or nystatin may be used.

If the otitis externa is *less severe* and there is little meatal swelling, it may respond to a combination of antibiotic and steroid ear drops. The antibiotics are usually those that are *not* given systemically. The antibiotics most commonly used are neomycin, gramicidin and framycetin. Remember that prolonged use may result in fungal infection or in sensitivity dermatitis.

Prevention of recurrence

Prevention of recurrence is not always possible; the patient should be advised to keep the ears dry, especially when washing the hair or showering. A large piece of cotton wool coated in Vaseline and placed in the concha is advisable, and if the patient is very keen to swim it is worthwhile investing in custom-made silicone rubber earplugs. The use of a proprietory preparation of spirit and acetic acid prophylactically after swimming is useful in reducing otitis externa. Equally important is the avoidance of scratching and poking the ears. Itching may be controlled with antihistamines given orally, especially at bedtime. If meatal stenosis predisposes to recurrent infection, meatoplasty (surgical enlargement of meatus) may be advisable.

NB. Do not make a diagnosis of otitis externa until you have satisfied your-self that the tympanic membrane is intact. If the ear fails to settle, look again and again to make sure that you are not dealing with a case of otitis media with a discharging perforation.

FURUNCULOSIS

Furunculosis of the external canal results from infection of a hair follicle and so must occur in the lateral part of the meatus. The organism is usually *Staphylococcus*; the pain is often out of proportion to the visible lesion.

SYMPTOMS

Pain

Pain is as severe as that of renal colic and the patient may need pethidine. The pain is made much worse by movement of the pinna or pressure on the tragus.

Deafness

Deafness is usually slight and due to meatal occlusion by the furuncle.

Signs

There is often no visible lesion but the introduction of an aural speculum causes intense pain. If the furuncle is larger, it will be seen as a red swelling in the outer meatus and there may be more than one furuncle present. At a more advanced stage, the furuncle will be seen to be pointing or may present as a fluctuant abscess.

TREATMENT

The insertion of a wick soaked in 10% ichthammol in glycerine (Glyc & Ic) is painful at the time but provides rapid relief. Flucloxacillin should be given parenterally for 24 h, followed by oral medication.

Analgesics are necessary; the patient will often need pethidine and is not fit for work.

Recurrent cases are not common—exclude diabetes and take a nasal swab in case the patient is a *Staphylococcus* carrier.

EXOSTOSES

Exostoses or small osteomata of the external auditory meatus are fairly common and usually bilateral. They are much more common in those who swim a lot in cold water, although the reason is not known.

There may be 2 or 3 little tumours arising in each bony meatus. They are sessile, hard, smooth, covered with very thin skin and when gently probed are often exquisitely sensitive. Their rate of growth is extremely slow and they may give rise to no symptoms, but if wax or debris accumulates between the tympanic membrane and the exostoses, its removal may tax the patience of the most skilled manipulator. In such cases, surgical removal of the exostoses may be indicated and is carried out with the aid of the operating microscope and drill.

MALIGNANT DISEASE

Malignant disease of the auditory meatus is rare and usually occurs in the elderly. If confined to the outer meatus, it behaves like skin cancer and can be treated by wide excision and skin grafting. If it spreads to invade the middle ear, facial nerve and temporomandibular joint, it is a relentless and terrible affliction. Pain becomes intractable and intolerable and there is a blood-stained discharge from the ear.

Treatment then is by radiotherapy, radical surgery or a combination of the two. Treatment is not possible in some cases, and the outlook is poor in the extreme.

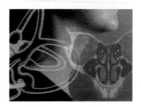

CHAPTER 7

Injury of the Tympanic Membrane

The tympanic membrane, being deeply placed, is well protected from injury. Damage does occur, however, and may be direct or indirect.

Direct trauma is caused by poking in the ear with sharp implements, such as hair grips, in an attempt to clean the ear; it is caused by syringing or unskilled attempts to remove wax or foreign bodies.

Indirect trauma is usually caused by pressure from a slap with an open hand or from blast injury; it may occur from temporal bone fracture (Fig. 7.1).

Welding sparks may cause severe damage to the tympanic membrane.

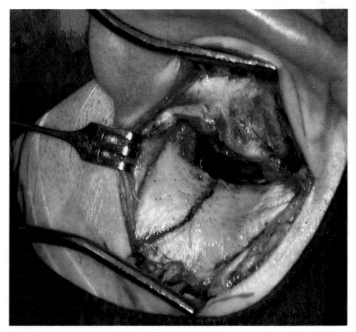

Fig. 7.1 Operative picture showing fracture of the temporal bone (which had caused facial nerve damage).

TEAR IN THE TYMPANIC MEMBRANE

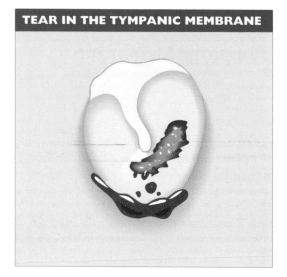

Fig. 7.2 Traumatic perforation of the tympanic membrane, showing a ragged perforation with blood in the external auditory canal.

SYMPTOMS

1   Pain, acute at time of rupture, usually transient.
2   Deafness, not usually severe, conductive in type. Cochlear damage may occur from excessive movement of the stapes.
3   Tinnitus, may be persistent — this is cochlear damage.
4   Vertigo, rarely.

SIGNS

1   Bleeding from the ear.
2   Blood clot in the meatus.
3   A visible tear in the tympanic membrane (Fig. 7.2).

TREATMENT — leave it alone

1   Do *not* clean out the ear.
2   Do *not* put in drops.
3   Do *not* syringe.

If the injury has been caused by direct trauma, treat with prophylactic antibiotics. In other cases, give antibiotics if there is evidence of infection supervening.

In virtually every case, the tear in the tympanic membrane will close rapidly. Do not regard the ear as healed until the hearing has returned to normal.

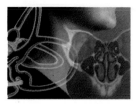

CHAPTER 8

Acute Otitis Media

Acute otitis media, i.e. acute inflammation of the middle-ear cavity, is a common condition and is frequently bilateral. It occurs most commonly in children and it is important that it is managed with care to prevent subsequent complications.

It most commonly follows an acute upper respiratory tract infection and may be viral or bacterial. Unless the ear discharges pus from which an organism is cultured it is impossible to decide one way or the other.

PATHOLOGY

Acute otitis media is an infection of the mucous membrane of the whole of the middle-ear cleft—Eustachian tube, tympanic cavity, attic, aditus, mastoid antrum and air cells.

The bacteria responsible for acute otitis media are: *Streptococcus pneumoniae* 35%, *Haemophilus influenzae* 25%, *Moraxella catarrhalis* 15%. Group A streptococci and *Staphylococcus aureus* may also be responsible.

The sequence of events in acute otitis media is as follows:

1 organisms invade the mucous membrane causing inflammation, oedema, exudate and later, pus;
2 oedema closes the Eustachian tube, preventing aeration and drainage;
3 pressure from the pus rises, causing the drum to bulge;
4 necrosis of the tympanic membrane results in perforation;
5 the ear continues to drain until the infection resolves.

CAUSES OF ACUTE OTITIS MEDIA

More common	Less common
Common cold	Sinusitis
Acute tonsillitis	Haemotympanum
Influenza	Trauma to the tympanic
Coryza of measles, scarlet fever, whooping cough	membrane
	Barotrauma (air flight)
	Diving
	Temporal bone fracture

Box 8.1 Causes of acute otitis media.

SYMPTOMS

Earache

Earache may be slight in a mild case, but more usually it is throbbing and severe. The child may cry and scream inconsolably until the ear perforates, the pain is relieved and peace is restored.

Deafness

Deafness is always present in acute otitis media. It is conductive in nature and may be accompanied by tinnitus. In an adult, the deafness or tinnitus may be the first complaint.

SIGNS

Pyrexia

The child is flushed and ill. The temperature may be as high as 40°C.

Tenderness

There is usually some tenderness to pressure on the mastoid antrum.

The tympanic membrane

The tympanic membrane varies in appearance according to the stage of the infection.

1 Loss of lustre and break-up of the light reflex.
2 Injection of the small vessels around the periphery and along the handle of the malleus.
3 Redness and fullness of the drum; the malleus handle becomes more vertical.
4 Bulging, with loss of landmarks. Purple colour. Outer layer may desquamate, causing blood-stained serous discharge. Early necrosis may be recognized, heralding imminent perforation.
5 Perforation with otorrhoea, which will often be blood-stained. Profuse and mucoid at first, later becoming thick and yellow.

Mucoid discharge

Mucoid discharge from an ear must mean that there is a perforation of the tympanic membrane. There are no mucous glands in the external canal.

TREATMENT

The treatment depends on the stage reached by the infection. The following stages may be considered: early, bulging and discharging.

Early

Antibiotics
Penicillin remains the drug of choice in most cases, and ideally should be given initially by injection followed by oral medication. In children under 5 years, when *Haemophilus influenzae* is likely to be present, amoxycillin will be more effective, and should always be considered if there is not a rapid response to penicillin. Co-amoxiclav is useful in Moraxella infections. Be guided by sensitivity reports from the laboratory.

Analgesics
Simple analgesics, such as aspirin or paracetamol, should suffice. Avoid the use of aspirin in children because of the risk of Reye's syndrome.

Nasal vasoconstrictors
The role of 0.5% ephedrine nasal drops is traditional but its value is uncertain in the presence of acute inflammation of the middle ear.

Ear drops
Ear drops are of no value in acute otitis media with an intact drum. Especially illogical is the use of drops containing local anaesthetics, which can have no effect on the middle-ear mucosa yet may cause a sensitivity reaction in the meatal skin.

Bulging

Myringotomy is necessary when bulging of the tympanic membrane persists, despite *adequate* antibiotic therapy. It should be carried out under general anaesthesia in theatre and a large incision in the membrane should be made to allow the ear to drain. Pus should be sent for bacteriological assessment.

Following myringotomy, the ear will discharge and the outer meatus should be dry-mopped regularly.

Discharging — nature's myringotomy

If the ear is already discharging when the patient is first seen, a swab should be sent for culture of the organism. Antibiotic therapy should be started but modified if necessary when the result of the sensitivities is known. Regular aural toilet will be necessary.

FURTHER MANAGEMENT

Do not consider acute otitis media to be cured until the hearing and the appearance of the membrane have returned to normal.

If resolution does not occur, suspect:

1 the nose, sinuses or nasopharynx? Infection may be present;
2 the choice or dose of antibiotic;
3 low-grade infection in the mastoid cells.

RECURRENT ACUTE OTITIS MEDIA (AOM)

Some children are susceptible to repeated attacks of AOM. There may be an underlying immunological deficit such as IgA deficiency or hypogamma-globulinaemia that will need to be investigated. Long-term treatment with half-dose cotrimoxazole may be beneficial. If the attacks persist, grommet insertion may prevent further attacks but may result in purulent discharge.

CHAPTER 9

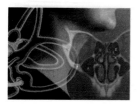

Chronic Otitis Media

If an attack of acute otitis media fails to heal, the perforation and discharge may in some cases persist. This leads to mixed infection and further damage to the middle-ear structures, with worsening conductive deafness. The predisposing factors in the development of chronic suppurative otitis media (CSOM) are listed in Box 9.1.

CAUSES OF CHRONIC OTITIS MEDIA:

1 Late treatment of acute otitis media.
2 Inadequate or inappropriate antibiotic therapy.
3 Upper airway sepsis.
4 Lowered resistance, e.g. malnutrition, anaemia, immunological impairment.
5 Particularly virulent infection, e.g. measles.

There are two major types of CSOM.
1 *Mucosal disease* with tympanic membrane perforation (tubo-tympanic disease, relatively safe).
2 *Bony*:
    (a) osteitis;
    (b) cholesteatoma—dangerous (attico-antral disease).

Box 9.1 Causes of chronic otitis media.

Mucosal infection

In these cases there may be underlying nasal or pharyngeal sepsis that will require attention if the ear is to heal. The ear will discharge, usually copiously, and the discharge is mucoid.

Remember—mucoid discharge from an ear must mean that there is a perforation present, even if you cannot identify it.

The perforation is in the pars tensa, and may be large or very small and difficult to see (Fig. 9.1).

Serious complications are very rare but if left untreated the condition may result in permanent deafness.

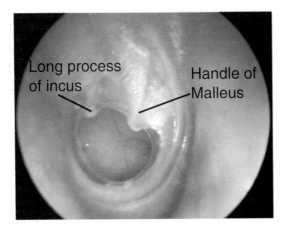

Fig. 9.1 A large central perforation of the tympanic membrane. The handle of the malleus and the long process of the incus are visible. (Courtesy of MPJ Yardley.)

The ear may become quiescent from time to time, a feature less likely to happen with bony CSOM, and the perforation may heal. If healing does not occur, surgical repair may be necessary.

TREATMENT OF MUCOSAL-TYPE CSOM

Ear discharge

When the ear is discharging, a swab should be sent for bacteriological analysis. The mainstay of treatment is thorough and regular aural toilet. Appropriate (as determined by the culture report) antibiotic therapy is instituted and in most cases the ear will rapidly become dry. The perforation may heal, especially if it is small. If the ear does not rapidly become dry, admission to hospital for regular aural toilet is often effective. If infection persists, look for chronic nasal or pharyngeal infection.

Dry perforation

When there is a dry perforation, surgery may be considered but is *not mandatory. Myringoplasty* is the repair of a tympanic membrane perforation; the tympanic membrane is exposed by an external incision, the rim of the perforation is stripped of epithelium and a graft is applied, usually on the medial aspect of the membrane. Various tissues have been used for graft material but that in most common use is autologous temporalis fascia, which is readily available at the operation site. Success rates for this procedure are very high; repair of the tympanic membrane may be combined with ossicular reconstruction, if necessary, in order to restore hearing — the operation is then referred to as a *tympanoplasty*.

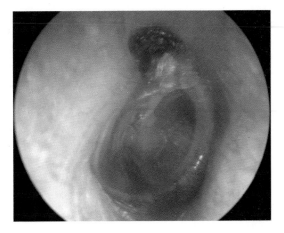

Fig. 9.2 Crusting of the pars flaccida suggestive of underlying cholesteatoma. (Courtesy of MPJ Yardley.)

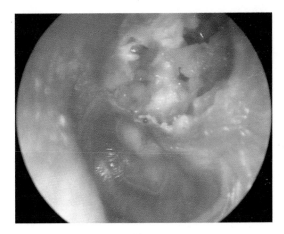

Fig. 9.3 Erosion of the attic bone to reveal cholesteatoma. (Courtesy of MPJ Yardley.)

BONY OR ATTICO-ANTRAL TYPE OF CSOM

The bone affected by this type of CSOM comprises the tympanic ring, the ossicles, the mastoid air cells and the bony walls of the attic, aditus and antrum. The perforation is postero-superior (Fig. 9.2) or in the pars flaccida (Schrapnell's membrane) (Fig. 9.3) and involves the bony annulus. The discharge is often scanty but usually persistent, and is often foul smelling.

There are other features of this type of CSOM.

1   Granulations as a result of osteitis—bright red and bleed on touch.

2   Aural polyps—formed of granulation tissue, which may fill the meatus and present at its outer end.

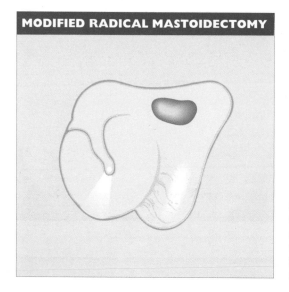

MODIFIED RADICAL MASTOIDECTOMY

Fig. 9.4 Modified radical mastoidectomy; note the shape of the cavity, the facial nerve ridge and the bulge caused by the lateral semicircular canal.

3 Cholesteatoma. This is formed by squamous epithelium within the middle-ear cleft, starting as a retraction pocket in the tympanic membrane. It results in accumulation of keratotic debris. This will be visible through the perforation as keratin flakes, which are white and smelly. The cholesteatoma expands and damages vital structures, such as dura, lateral sinus, facial nerve and lateral semicircular canal. *Cholesteatoma is potentially lethal if untreated.*

TREATMENT OF BONY-TYPE CSOM

1 Regular aural toilet in early cases of annular osteitis may be adequate to prevent progression, but such a case should be watched closely.

2 Suction toilet under the microscope may evacuate a small pocket of cholesteatoma, and a dry ear may result.

3 *Mastoidectomy* is nearly always necessary in established cholesteatoma and takes several forms, depending on the extent of the disease (Fig. 9.4).

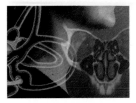

CHAPTER 10

Complications of Middle-Ear Infection

Acute mastoiditis

Acute mastoiditis is the result of extension of acute otitis media into the mastoid air cells with suppuration and bone necrosis. Common in the preantibiotic era, it is now rare in the Western world (Fig. 10.1).

SYMPTOMS

1 Pain—persistent and throbbing.
2 Otorrhoea—usually creamy and profuse.
3 Increasing deafness.

SIGNS

1 Pyrexia.
2 General state—the patient is obviously ill.
3 Tenderness is marked over the mastoid antrum.
4 Swelling in the postauricular region, with obliteration of the sulcus. The pinna is pushed down and forward (Fig. 10.2).
5 Sagging of the meatal roof or posterior wall.
6 The tympanic membrane is either perforated and the ear discharging, or it is red and bulging.
If the tympanic membrane is normal, the patient does not have acute mastoiditis.

INVESTIGATIONS

1 White blood count—raised neutrophil count.
2 CT scanning shows opacity and air cell coalescence.

OCCASIONAL FEATURES OF ACUTE MASTOIDITIS

1 Subperiosteal abscess over the mastoid process.
2 Bezold's abscess—pus breaks through the mastoid tip and forms an abscess in the neck.
3 Zygomatic mastoiditis—results in swelling over the zygoma.

CHRONIC OTITIS MEDIA

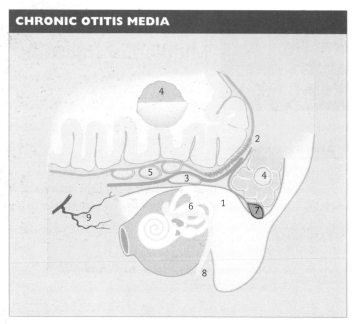

Fig. 10.1 Complications of chronic otitis media. 1, Acute mastoiditis; 2, Meningitis; 3, Extradural abscess; 4, Brain abscess (temporal lobe and cerebellum); 5, Subdural abscess; 6, Labyrinthitis; 7, Lateral sinus thrombosis; 8, Facial nerve paralysis; 9, Petrositis.

TREATMENT

When the diagnosis of acute mastoiditis has been made, do not delay. The patient should be admitted to hospital.

1 Antibiotics should be administered intravenously (i.v). The choice of antibiotic, as always, depends on the sensitivity of the organism. If the organism is not known and there is no pus to culture, start amoxycillin and metronidazole immediately.

2 Cortical mastoidectomy. If there is a subperiosteal abscess or if the response to antibiotics is not rapid and complete, cortical mastoidectomy must be performed. The mastoid is exposed by a postaural incision and the cortex is removed by drilling. All mastoid air cells are then opened, removing pus and granulations. The incision is closed with drainage. The object of this operation is to drain the mastoid antrum and air cells but leave the middle ear, the ossicles and the external meatus untouched.

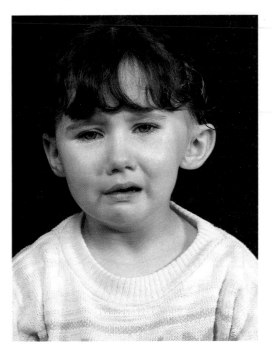

Fig. 10.2 Acute mastoiditis.

Meningitis

CLINICAL FEATURES

1 The patient is unwell.
2 Pyrexia — may only be slight.
3 Neck rigidity.
4 Positive Kernig's sign.
5 Photophobia.
6 Cerebrospinal fluid (CSF) — lumbar puncture essential unless there is raised intracranial pressure (q.v).
    (a) Often cloudy.
    (b) Pressure raised.
    (c) White cells raised.
    (d) Protein raised.
    (e) Chloride lowered.
    (f) Glucose lowered.
    (g) Organisms present on culture and Gram stain.

TREATMENT

1   Do not give antibiotic until CSF has been obtained for culture and confirmation of diagnosis. Then start penicillin parenterally and intrathecally.

2   Mastoidectomy is necessary if meningitis results from mastoiditis and should not be delayed. The type of operation will be dictated by the extent and nature of the ear disease.

Extradural abscess

An abscess formed by direct extension either above the tegmen or around the lateral sinus (perisinus abscess).

The features of mastoiditis are present and often accentuated. Severe pain is common. The condition may only be recognized at operation.

In addition to antibiotics, mastoid surgery is essential to treat the underlying ear disease and drain the abscess.

Brain abscess

Otogenic brain abscess may occur in the cerebellum or in the temporal lobe of the cerebrum. The two routes by which infection reaches the brain are by direct spread via bone and meninges or via blood vessels, i.e. thrombophlebitis.

A brain abscess may develop with great speed or may develop more gradually over a period of months. The effects are produced by:

1   systemic effects of infection, i.e. malaise, pyrexia — which may be absent;

2   raised intracranial pressure, i.e. headache, drowsiness, confusion, impaired consciousness, papilloedema;

3   localizing signs.

TEMPORAL LOBE ABSCESS

Localizing signs (Fig. 10.3):

1   dysphasia — more common with left-sided abscesses;

2   contralateral upper quadrantic homonymous hemianopia;

3   paralysis — contralateral face and arm, rarely leg;

4   hallucinations of taste and smell.

CEREBELLAR ABSCESS

Localizing signs:

1   neck stiffness;

2   weakness and loss of tone on same side;

3   ataxia — falling to same side;

4   intention tremor with past-pointing;

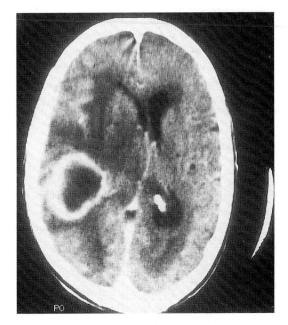

Fig. 10.3 CT scan with contrast showing temporal lobe abscess resulting from chronic middle ear disease. (Courtesy of Dr T. Hodgson.)

5 dysdiadokokinesis;

6 nystagmus — coarse and slow;

7 vertigo — sometimes.

DIAGNOSIS OF INTRACRANIAL SEPSIS:

1 Any patient with chronic ear disease who develops pain or headache should be suspected of having intracranial extension.

2 Any patient who has otogenic meningitis, labyrinthitis or lateral sinus thrombosis may also have a brain abscess.

3 Lumbar puncture may be dangerous owing to pressure coning.

4 Neurosurgical advice should be sought at an early stage if intracranial suppuration is suspected.

5 Confirmation and localization of the abscess will require further investigation.

Computerized tomography (CT) scanning will demonstrate intracranial abscesses reliably and should always be performed when it is suspected. Magnetic resonance (MR) imaging shows soft-tissue lesions with more detail than CT but gives no bone detail. If in doubt what to do, discuss the problem with a radiologist.

TREATMENT

It is the brain abscess that will kill the patient, and it is this that must take surgical priority. The abscess should be drained through a burr hole, or excised via a craniotomy and then, if the patient's condition permits, mastoidectomy should be performed under the same anaesthetic. After pus has been obtained for culture, aggressive therapy with antibiotics is essential, to be amended as necessary when the sensitivity is known.

PROGNOSIS

The prognosis of brain abscess has improved with the use of antibiotics and modern diagnostic methods but still carries a high mortality; the outlook is better for cerebral abscesses than cerebellar, in which the mortality rate may be 70%. Left untreated, death from brain abscess occurs from pressure coning, rupture into a ventricle or spreading encephalitis.

Subdural abscess

Subdural abscess more commonly occurs in the frontal region from sinusitis, but may result from ear disease. Focal epilepsy may develop from cortical damage. The prognosis is poor.

Labyrinthitis

Infection may reach the labyrinth by erosion of a fistula by cholesteatoma. It may rarely arise in acute otitis media.

CLINICAL FEATURES

1   Vertigo may be mild in serous labyrinthitis or overwhelming in purulent labyrinthitis.
2   Nausea and vomiting.
3   Nystagmus towards the opposite side.
4   There may be a positive *fistula test*—pressure on the tragus causes vertigo or eye deviation by inducing movement of the perilymph.
5   There will be profound sensorineural deafness in purulent labyrinthitis.

TREATMENT

1   Antibiotics.
2   Mastoidectomy for chronic ear disease.
3   Occasionally, labyrinthine drainage.

Lateral sinus thrombosis

A perisinus abscess from mastoiditis causes thrombosis of the lateral sinus and ascending cortical thrombo-phlebitis. Septic emboli are given off and metastatic abscesses may occur. The prognosis is poor but improved by early diagnosis and treatment.

CLINICAL FEATURES

1   Swinging pyrexia — up to 40 °C.
2   Rigors.
3   Polymorph leucocytosis.
4   Positive Tobey–Ayer test — sometimes. Compression of contralateral internal jugular vein → rise in CSF pressure. Compression of ipsilateral internal jugular vein → no rise.
5   Meningeal signs — sometimes.
6   Positive blood cultures, especially if taken during a rigor.
7   Papilloedema — sometimes.
8   Metastatic abscesses — prognosis poor.
9   Cortical signs — facial weakness, hemiparesis.

TREATMENT

1   Antibiotics.
2   Mastoidectomy with wide exposure of the lateral sinus and even removal of infected thrombus.

Facial paralysis

Facial paralysis can result from both acute and chronic otitis media.
1   Acute otitis media — especially in children and especially if the facial nerve canal in the middle ear is dehiscent. It is, however, uncommon.
2   Chronic otitis media — cholesteatoma may erode the bone around the horizontal and vertical parts of the facial nerve, and infection and granulations cause facial paralysis.
In the early stages, the patient will complain of dribbling from the corner of the mouth. Clinical examination confirms the diagnosis — it may be difficult to detect if the weakness is minimal.

TREATMENT

If due to acute otitis media, a full recovery with antibiotic therapy is to be expected.

If due to CSOM, mastoidectomy is mandatory, with clearance of disease from around the facial nerve.

Remember — a facial palsy occurring in the presence of chronic ear disease is **not** Bell's palsy and active treatment is needed if the palsy is not to become permanent. *Do not give steroids.*

Petrositis

Very rarely, infection may spread to the petrous apex and involve the VIth cranial nerve.

CLINICAL FEATURES (GRADENIGO'S SYNDROME):

1. Diplopia from lateral rectus palsy.
2. Trigeminal pain.
3. Evidence of middle-ear infection.

TREATMENT

1. Antibiotics.
2. Mastoidectomy with drainage of the apical cells.

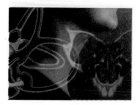

CHAPTER 11

Otitis Media with Effusion

Otitis media with effusion (OME), or 'glue ear', is a present-day epidemic affecting up to one-third of all children at some time in their lives. The condition is due to the accumulation of fluid, either serous or viscous, within the middle-ear cleft, resulting in conductive deafness. It is commonest in small children and those of primary school age and may cause significant deafness. It is essential that general practitioners are able to recognize the condition. It may be responsible for developmental and educational impairment, and if untreated may result in permanent middle-ear changes. It occurs in adults, usually as a serous effusion and may rarely be a sign of nasopharyngeal malignancy.

SYMPTOMS

1 Deafness may be the only symptom.
2 Discomfort in the ear — rarely severe.
3 Occasionally, tinnitus or unsteadiness.

CAUSES OF OME

1 Nasopharyngeal obstruction, e.g. large adenoids or tumour resulting in Eustachian tube dysfunction. The condition may be associated with recurrent attacks of acute otitis media.
2 Acute otitis media, untreated, will often give rise to a spontaneous perforation and drainage of the middle ear. Such a result will be prevented by treatment with an antibiotic and, if treatment is inadequate, middle-ear effusion may occur.
3 Allergic rhinitis, often missed in children, will predispose to middle-ear effusions.
4 Parental smoking has been shown to predispose to OME in children.
5 OME is commoner in winter months.
6 Otitic barotrauma — most commonly caused by descent in an aircraft, especially if the subject has a cold. Failure of middle-ear ventilation results in middle-ear effusion, sometimes blood-stained. Also occurs in scuba divers.
7 In many cases of secretory otitis media, no cause is apparent.

Box 11.1 Causes of otitis media with effusion.

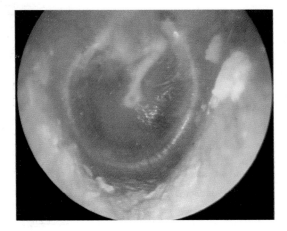

Fig. 11.1 Otitis media with effusion. Note the yellow discoloration of the tympanic membrane. (Courtesy of MPJ Yardley.)

SIGNS

1 Fluid in the middle ear—a variable appearance that may be difficult to recognize.

2 Dull appearance with radial vessels visible on the tympanic membrane and handle of the malleus.

3 Retraction of the tympanic membrane.

4 Yellow/orange tinge to tympanic membrane (Fig. 11.1) *or*

5 Dark blue or grey colour of tympanic membrane.

6 Hair lines or bubbles—rarely seen.

7 Tuning fork tests show conductive deafness, i.e. bone conduction > air conduction

8 Flat impedance curve.

TREATMENT

In children

1 Many cases will resolve spontaneously, and the child should usually be observed for 3 months before embarking on surgery.

2 The use of antihistamines and mucolytics is of no proven benefit. Antibiotic therapy may help in the short term. Surgery is indicated if hearing loss persists for 3 months or if there is recurring pain.

3 Surgical treatment.

Adenoidectomy

It has been shown that adenoidectomy is beneficial in the long-term resolution of OME. The maximum benefit occurs between the ages of 4 and 8 years.

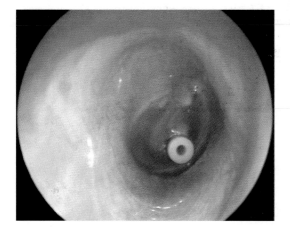

Fig. 11.2 Right tympanic membrane with grommet in place. (Courtesy of MPJ Yardley.)

Myringotomy and grommet insertion (Fig. 11.2)

Myringotomy and grommet insertion is now the most commonly performed operation in the UK and USA. Under general anaesthetic, the tympanic membrane is incised antero-inferiorly. The glue is aspirated and a grommet inserted into the incision. The function of the grommet is to ventilate the middle ear and not to drain the fluid; most surgeons now allow swimming after grommet insertion, but not diving or swimming under water. The grommet will extrude after a variable period, the average time being 6 months. Repeated insertion is sometimes necessary if the effusion recurs.

In adults

Examination of the nasopharynx to exclude tumour is essential, especially if the effusion is unilateral. Under the same anaesthetic, a grommet may be inserted.

Secretory otitis media in adults not due to tumour usually follows a cold. Resolution is usually spontaneous, but may take up to 6 weeks.

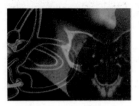

CHAPTER 12

Otosclerosis

Otosclerosis, usually an hereditary disorder, causes abnormal bone to be formed around the stapes footplate, preventing its normal movement. Conductive deafness then results. More rarely, the bone of the cochlea is affected and results in sensorineural deafness.

CLINICAL FEATURES OF OTOSCLEROSIS

1 Usual onset in second and third decades.
2 Two-thirds give a family history.
3 Two-thirds are female. The gene is not sex-linked but pregnancy may make the deafness worse. Not many men get pregnant, so more females present for treatment!
4 Deafness may be unilateral or bilateral.
5 Paracusis is often present—the patient is able to hear better in noisy surroundings.
6 Tinnitus is often present—it may not be relieved by operation.
7 The tympanic membranes are normal.
8 Tuning fork tests show the deafness to be conductive.
9 Cochlear impairment may be present.
10 Audiometry. Air conduction impaired. Bone conduction initially normal but deteriorates as the disease progresses.

Box 12.1 Clinical features of otosclerosis.

TREATMENT

Stapedectomy

First performed in 1956, stapedectomy is an elegant solution to the problem. The middle ear is exposed (Fig. 12.1), the stapes superstructure is removed and the footplate perforated. A prosthesis of stainless steel or Teflon in place of the stapes is attached to the long process of the incus with its distal end in the oval window (Fig. 12.2). The patient is usually discharged the following day and should refrain from strenuous activity for at least a month. Stapedectomy may result in total loss of hearing in the operated ear, and patients should be made aware of such risk *before* operation.

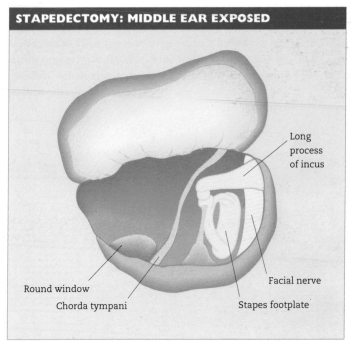

STAPEDECTOMY: MIDDLE EAR EXPOSED

Long process of incus

Round window

Chorda tympani

Facial nerve

Stapes footplate

Fig. 12.1 The surgical approach to stapedectomy, showing the tympano-meatal flap elevated.

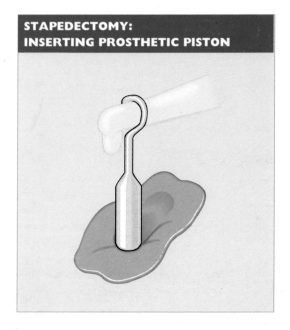

STAPEDECTOMY: INSERTING PROSTHETIC PISTON

Fig. 12.2 Stapedectomy. The superstructure of the stapes has been removed, the footplate opened and covered with a vein before inserting a prosthetic piston.

Hearing aids and lip-reading

Modern hearing aids are of great benefit to patients with conductive deafness and have the advantage of causing no risk to the patient's hearing. A hearing aid should always be offered to a patient as an alternative to surgery. If the disease is progressing rapidly and profound deafness seems likely, instruction in lip-reading should never be neglected at a stage when the patient still has usable hearing.

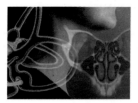

CHAPTER 13

Earache (Otalgia)

Earache may be due to ear disease, or may be referred from disease elsewhere. It is referred earache that so often causes difficulty in diagnosis.

Aural causes

Earache may be caused by any disease of the external ear or middle-ear cleft and the diagnosis is obvious on examination of the ear. The most common causes are *acute otitis media*, *acute otitis externa*, *furunculosis* and, very rarely, *acute mastoiditis*. Malignant disease of the ear will cause intractable earache. If the ear is not convincingly abnormal, look for a source of referred otalgia; you will nearly always find it.

Referred earache

Pain may be referred to the ear via the following nerves:

1   **the auriculo-temporal branch of the trigeminal nerve** from, for example, carious teeth, impacted molar teeth, the temporomandibular joint or the tongue;

2   **tympanic branch of the glossopharyngeal nerve** from, for example, tonsillectomy, tonsillitis/quinsy, carcinoma of base of tongue or tonsil or glosso-pharyngeal neuralgia;

3   **sensory branch of the facial nerve** from, for example, herpes zoster;

4   **auricular branch of the vagus nerve** from, for example, carcinoma of larynx, carcinoma of piriform fossa or postcricoid carcinoma;

5   **great auricular nerve (C2–3) and lesser occipital nerve (C2)** from, for example, cervical spondylosis.

Some causes of referred otalgia merit special mention on account of their frequency or diagnostic importance.

POST-TONSILLECTOMY EARACHE

Post-tonsillectomy earache is usual, but do not forget to examine the ear. Otitis media may be present.

TEMPOROMANDIBULAR JOINT DYSFUNCTION

Temporomandibular joint dysfunction or pain dysfunction syndrome is common and often not diagnosed. There may be severe earache, trismus and a feeling of fullness in the ear. It is sometimes associated with faulty dental occlusion but is often simply due to grinding or clenching the teeth. There is tenderness and clicking of the temporomandibular joint and tenderness of the medial pterygoid muscle intraorally. *Advice*: a bite-raising splint, soft diet and correction of malocclusion are usually curative.

MALIGNANT DISEASE

Malignant disease of the posterior tongue, vallecula, tonsil, larynx or pharynx often produces earache, which may be an early symptom. The combination of earache with dysphagia, especially if there is an enlarged cervical node, means cancer until proved otherwise.

NB. The problem of referred earache is often misdiagnosed through lack of thought. If the earache has no obvious aural cause, look for a source of referred pain.

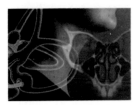

CHAPTER 14

Tinnitus

Tinnitus, the complaint of noises in the ears, is common and difficult to relieve. The tinnitus may be constant or intermittent and usually varies in its intensity and character. It is more apparent in quiet surroundings and is aggravated by fatigue, anxiety and depression. It is not a disease but a symptom.

MANAGEMENT

The management of tinnitus is a severe test of a doctor's art because so often little can be done to eliminate it. However, several points will be helpful as a guide.

1   Take the patient's fears and complaints seriously and obtain a thorough history.

2   Examination of the patient should also be thorough. A quick look at the tympanic membranes is only a gesture.

3   If an abnormality of the ear, such as impacted wax or serous otitis media, is found, treatment will often cure the tinnitus.

4   Tinnitus due to chronic degeneration, such as presbycusis, ototoxity or noise-induced deafness, is usually permanent in some degree and it is dishonest to suggest that one day it will disappear. The patient will become increasingly disappointed. It is far better that the patient understands the nature of the condition and, with time, the tinnitus will obtrude less as he or she adjusts to it and avoids circumstances that aggravate it.

5   Many patients fear that tinnitus indicates serious disease of the ear or a brain tumour. Reassurance will be more credible if examination of the patient has been adequate.

6   Drug treatment, such as sedatives and antidepressants, may help the patient but will not eliminate tinnitus. Anticonvulsant drugs and vasodilators occasionally may be of benefit but their effectiveness cannot be predicted.

7   Patients with depression are particularly susceptible to the effects of tinnitus and it should be treated thoroughly and expertly.

8   If the patient with tinnitus is also deaf, a hearing aid is very helpful in masking the tinnitus as well as in relieving the deafness, and many patients are very grateful for this simple advice.

9   Tinnitus maskers, by producing white noise, will also make tinnitus less obtrusive. The masking device looks like a postaural hearing aid and its output characteristics can be adjusted to obtain the most effective masking.

10   If the patient is kept awake by tinnitus, a radio with a time switch may help.

11   Relaxation techniques have been found to be helpful by many patients.

12   Acupuncture and herbal remedies are of unproved value in tinnitus.

LOCAL AND GENERAL CAUSES OF TINNITUS

Local causes

Tinnitus may be a symptom of any abnormal condition of the ear and may be associated with any form of deafness. Certain conditions deserve special mention:

1   presbycusis — often causes tinnitus;

2   Menière's disease — tinnitus is usually worse with the acute attacks;

3   noise-induced deafness — tinnitus may be worse immediately after exposure to noise;

4   otosclerosis?; tinnitus may be relieved by stapedectomy but should not be the major indication for surgery;

5   glomus jugulare tumour — tinnitus is pulsating and may be audible through a stethoscope;

6   aneurysm, vascular malfomation and some vascular intracranial tumours can also cause tinnitus, which may even be heard by an examiner.

General causes

Tinnitus is often a feature of general ill-health as, for example, in:

1   fever of any cause;

2   cardiovascular disease — hypertension, atheroma, cardiac failure;

3   blood disease — anaemia, raised viscosity;

4   neurological disease — multiple sclerosis, neuropathy;

5   drug treatment — aspirin, quinine, ototoxic drugs;

6   alcohol abuse.

Box 14.1   Local and general causes of tinnitus.

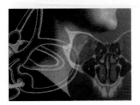

CHAPTER 15

Vertigo

Vertigo is a subjective sensation of movement, usually rotatory but sometimes linear. It is often accompanied by pallor, sweating and vomiting. The objective sign of vertigo is nystagmus.

Bodily balance is maintained by the input to the brain from the inner ear, the eyes and the proprioceptive organs, especially of the neck; dysfunction of any of these systems may lead to imbalance.

The diagnosis of the cause of vertigo or imbalance depends mostly on history, much on examination and little on investigation. The particular questions to be asked relate to three areas.

1　Timing: episodic, persistent.

2　Aural symptoms: deafness, fluctuating or progressive; tinnitus; earache; discharge.

3　Neurological symptoms: loss of consciousness; weakness; numbness; dysarthria; diplopia; fitting.

Table 15.1 gives a guide to diagnosis following history-taking and will direct any specific examination and investigation.

Menière's disease

Menière's disease is a condition of unknown aetiology in which there is distension of the membranous labyrinth by accumulation of endolymph. It can occur at any age, but its onset is most common between 40 and 60 years. It usually starts in one ear only, but in about 25% of cases the second ear becomes affected. The clinical features are as follows.

1　Vertigo is intermittent but may be profound, and usually causes vomiting. The vertigo rarely lasts for more than a few hours, and is of a rotational nature.

2　A feeling of fullness in the ear may precede an attack by hours or even days.

3　Deafness is sensorineural and is more severe before and during an attack. It is associated with distortion and loudness intolerance (recruitment). Despite fluctuations, the deafness is usually steadily progressive and may become severe.

4　Tinnitus is constant but more severe before an attack. It may precede all

GUIDE TO DIAGNOSIS OF VERTIGO

Episodic with aural symptoms
Menière's disease
Migraine

Episodic without aural symptoms
Benign paroxysmal positional vertigo
Migraine
Transient ischaemic attacks
Epilepsy
Cardiac arrhythmia
Postural hypotension
Cervical spondylosis

Constant with aural symptoms
Chronic otitis media with labyrinthine fistula
Ototoxicity
Acoustic neuroma

Constant without aural symptoms
Multiple sclerosis
Posterior fossa tumour
Cardiovascular disease
Degenerative disorder of the vestibular labyrinth
Hyperventilation
Alcoholism

Solitary acute attack with aural symptoms
Head injury
Labyrinthine fistula
Viral infection, e.g. mumps, herpes zoster
Vascular occlusion
Round-window membrane rupture

Solitary acute attack without aural symptoms
Vasovagal faint
Vestibular neuronitis
Trauma

Table 15.1 Guide to diagnosis of vertigo.

other symptoms by many months, and its cause only becomes apparent later.

TREATMENT

General and medical measures

In an acute attack, when vomiting is likely to occur, oral medication is of limited value, but cinnarizine, 15–30 mg 6-hourly, or prochlorperazine,

5–10 mg 6-hourly, are useful preparations. Alternatively, prochlorperazine can be given as a suppository or sublabially, or chlorpromazine (25 mg) may be given as an intramuscular injection.

Between attacks, various methods of treatment are useful.

1 Fluid and salt restriction.

2 Avoidance of smoking and excessive alcohol or coffee.

3 Regular therapy with betahistine hydrochloride, 8–16 mg t.d.s.

4 If the attacks are frequent, regular medication with labyrinthine sedatives, such as cinnarizine, 15–30 mg t.d.s., or prochlorperazine, 5–10 mg t.d.s., are of value. Regular low-dose diuretic therapy may also be of benefit.

Surgical treatment

1 Labyrinthectomy is effective in relieving vertigo, but should only be performed in the unilateral case and when the hearing is already severely impaired.

2 Drainage of the endolymphatic sac by the transmastoid route.

3 Division of the vestibular nerve either by the middle fossa or by the retrolabyrinthine route; this operation preserves the hearing but is a more hazardous procedure.

4 Intra-tympanic gentamycin is helpful in reducing vestibular activity but with a 10% risk of worsening the hearing loss.

Ménière's disease is fortunately uncommon, but may be incapacitating. The patient requires constant reassurance and sympathetic support.

Vestibular neuronitis

Although occasionally epidemic, vestibular neuronitis is probably of viral origin and causes vestibular failure. The vertigo is usually of explosive onset, but there is neither tinnitus nor deafness. Steady resolution takes place over a period of 6–12 weeks but the acute phase usually clears in 2 weeks.

Benign paroxysmal positional vertigo

Benign paroxysmal positional vertigo is due to a degenerative condition of the utricular neuroepithelium and may occur spontaneously or following head injury. It is also seen in CSOM. Attacks of vertigo are precipitated by turning the head so that the affected ear is undermost; the vertigo occurs following a latent period of several seconds and is of brief duration. Nystagmus will be observed but repeated testing results in abolition of the vertigo. Steady resolution is to be expected over a period of weeks or months. It may be recurrent. It can often be relieved completely by the Epley manoeuvre of particle repositioning by sequential movement of the head to move the otolith particles away from the macula.

Vertebrobasilar insufficiency

Vertebrobasilar insufficiency may cause momentary attacks of vertigo pre-cipitated by neck extension, e.g. hanging washing on a line. The diagnosis is more certain if other evidence of brain stem ischaemia, such as dysarthria or diplopia, is also present. Severe ischaemia may cause drop attacks with-out loss of consciousness.

Ototoxic drugs

Ototoxic drugs, such as gentamycin and other aminoglycoside antibiotics, can cause disabling ataxia by destruction of labyrinthine function. Such atax-ia may be permanent and the risk is reduced by careful monitoring of serum levels of the drug, especially in patients with renal impairment. There is not usually any rotational vertigo.

Trauma to the labyrinth

Trauma to the labyrinth causing vertigo may complicate head injury, with or without temporal bone fracture.

Post-operative vertigo

Post-operative vertigo may occur after ear surgery, especially stapedec-tomy, and will usually settle in a few days.

Suppurative labyrinthitis

Suppurative labyrinthitis causes severe vertigo (see complications of middle-ear disease). It also results in a total loss of hearing.

Syphilitic labyrinthitis

Syphilitic labyrinthitis from acquired or congenital syphilis is very rare but may cause vertigo and/or progressive deafness. Do not forget the spirochaete.

Acoustic neuroma

Acoustic neuroma (vestibular schwannoma) is a slow-growing benign tumour of the vestibular nerve that causes hearing loss and slow loss of vestibular function. Imbalance rather than vertigo results.

Geniculate herpes zoster

Geniculate herpes zoster (Ramsay Hunt syndrome) usually causes vertigo, along with facial palsy and severe pain in the ear.

Perilymph fistula

As a result of spontaneous rupture of the round-window membrane or trauma to the stapes footplate, perilymph fistula causes marked vertigo with tinnitus and deafness. There is usually a history of straining, lifting or subaqua diving in the spontaneous cases, and treatment is by bed-rest initially, followed by surgical repair if symptoms persist.

CHAPTER 16

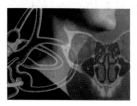

Facial Nerve Paralysis

Paralysis of the facial nerve is a subject of fascination to the otologist and a cause of distress to the patient. Owing to its frequency and diversity of aetiology, it is a matter of very considerable importance to workers in all spheres of medical life.

The causes are numerous and are considered in Table 16.1.

DIAGNOSIS

The patient presents with a varying degree of weakness of the facial muscles and sometimes difficulty in clearing food from the bucco gingival sulcus as a result of buccinator paralysis.

Facial asymmetry is accentuated by attempting to close the eyes tightly, to show the teeth or to whistle (Fig. 16.1).

It is important to remember that in **supranuclear lesions** the movements of the upper part of the face are likely to be unaffected as the forehead muscles have bilateral cortical representation. Moreover, involuntary movements (e.g. smiling) may be retained even in the lower face. A most careful history and aural and neurological examination are essential, including attention to such matters as impaired taste (lesion is above origin of chorda tympani), hyperacusis with loss of the stapedius reflex (lesion is above nerve to stapedius) or reduction of lacrimation (lesion is above geniculate ganglion).

Electrodiagnosis is used in the assessment of the degree of involvement of the nerve and includes nerve conduction tests and electromyography. A detailed description of the various tests is beyond the scope of this volume, but their application is of value as a guide to prognosis and management.

Bell's palsy (idiopathic facial paralysis)

Bell's palsy is a lower motor neurone facial palsy of unknown cause, but possibly viral. It is part of the group of idiopathic cranial mono-neuropathies. Bell's palsy may be complete or incomplete; the more severe the palsy, the worse the prognosis for recovery. In practice, full recovery may be expected in 85% of cases. The remainder may develop complications, such as ectropion or synkinesis.

CAUSES OF FACIAL NERVE PARALYSIS

Supranuclear and nuclear
Cerebral vascular lesions
Poliomyelitis
Cerebral tumours

Infranuclear
Bell's palsy
Trauma (birth injury, fractured temporal bone, surgical)
Tumours (acoustic neurofibroma, parotid tumours, malignant disease of the middle ear)
Suppuration (acute or chronic otitis media)
Ramsay Hunt syndrome
Multiple sclerosis
Guillain–Barré syndrome
Sarcoidosis

Table 16.1 Causes of facial nerve paralysis.

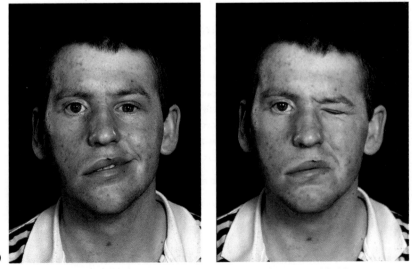

(b)

Fig. 16.1 Post-traumatic right facial palsy. Shown at rest (left) and on attempted eye closure.

TREATMENT

Treatment of Bell's palsy should not be delayed.

1   Prednisolone given orally is the treatment of choice, but only if started in the first 24h. In an adult, start with 80 mg daily and reduce the dose steadily to zero over a period of 2 weeks.

2   Surgical decompression of the facial nerve is a matter of controversy: some authorities decompress at an early stage: most do not advise decompression.

3   Tarsorrhaphy may be needed to protect the cornea of the unblinking eye.

4   In the rare event of recovery not taking place, cross-facial grafting or hypoglossal–facial anastomosis may be carried out to restore symmetry to the face.

5   Inward collapse of the cheek can be disguised with a built-up denture to restore the contour.

Do not make a diagnosis of Bell's palsy until you have excluded other causes. If recovery does not take place in 6 months, reconsider the diagnosis.

Ramsay Hunt syndrome

This is due to herpes zoster infection of the geniculate ganglion, affecting more rarely the IX and X nerves and, very occasionally, the V, VI or XII. The patient is usually elderly, and severe pain precedes the facial palsy and the herpetic eruption in the ear (sometimes on the tongue and palate). The patient usually has vertigo, and the hearing is impaired. Recovery of facial nerve function is much less likely than in Bell's palsy.

Prompt treatment with acyclovir given orally may improve the prognosis and reduce post-herpetic neuralgia.

Facial palsy in acute or chronic otitis media

This requires immediate expert advice, as urgent surgical treatment is usually necessary.

Traumatic facial palsy

This may result from fracture of the temporal bone or from ear surgery. If the onset is delayed, recovery is to be expected but if there is immediate palsy, urgent surgical exploration and decompression or grafting will be required. Otological advice should be sought without delay (Fig. 7.1).

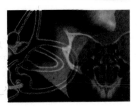

CHAPTER 17

Clinical Examination of the Nose and Nasopharynx

Most students are unaware of the interior dimensions of the nose, which extends horizontally backwards for 65–76 mm to the posterior choanae. The inside of the nose may be obscured by mucosal oedema, septal deviations or polyps and only with practice is adequate visualization possible.

The first requirement is adequate lighting. Ideally this is obtained with a head-mirror, but a bright torch or auriscope provide reasonable alternatives.

Anterior rhinoscopy

Anterior rhinoscopy is carried out with Thudichum's speculum (Fig. 17.1), which is introduced gently into the nose. The nasal mucosa is very sensitive! In children, a speculum is often not necessary as an adequate view can be obtained by lifting the nasal tip with the thumb.

On looking into the nose the anterior septum and inferior turbinates are easily seen (Fig. 17.2). It is a common error to mistake the turbinates for a nasal polyp. If you examine enough noses, you will not make that mistake.

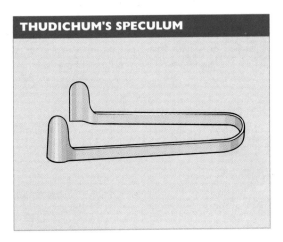

THUDICHUM'S SPECULUM

Fig. 17.1 Thudichum's speculum.

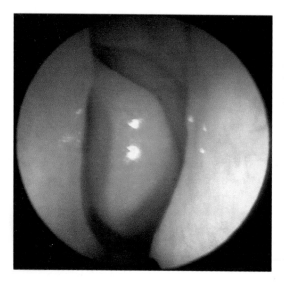

Fig. 17.2 The appearance of the normal nose showing the inferior turbinate attached to the lateral nasal wall. (Courtesy of TJ Woolford.)

Nasal endoscope

Rigid or fibre-optic endoscopes have made examination of the nasopharynx much easier. The instrument is introduced through the nose and the postnasal space can be inspected at leisure. It has the advantage of allowing photography and simultaneous viewing by an observer. It also allows minute inspection of the nasal cavity.

Assessment of the nasal airway

Assessment of the nasal airway can be made easily by holding a cool polished surface, such as a metal tongue depressor, below the nostrils. The area of condensation from each side of the nose can be compared.

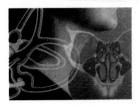

CHAPTER 18

Foreign Body in the Nose

Children between the ages of 1 and 4 years sometimes insert foreign bodies into one or both nostrils (Fig. 18.1). The objects of their choice may be hard, such as buttons, beads or ball bearings, or soft, such as paper, cotton wool, rubber or other vegetable materials; the latter, being as a rule more irritating, tend to give rise to symptoms more quickly.

The child, however intelligent, is unlikely to indicate that a foreign body is present in his nose; he may, in fact, deny the possibility in order to avoid rebuke. A sibling may give the game away.

CLINICAL FEATURES

1   A fretful child.
2   Unilateral evil-smelling nasal discharge, sometimes blood-stained.
3   Excoriation around the nostril.
4   Occasionally, X-ray evidence.

DANGERS

1   Injury from clumsy attempts at removal by unskilled persons.
2   Local spread of infection — sinusitis or meningitis.
3   Inhalation of foreign body — leading to lung collapse and infection.

MANAGEMENT

Casualty officers in particular should be alive to the possibility of nasal foreign bodies in small children. The child's mother may say that she suspects a foreign body, or the presence of a foreign body may be obvious. On the other hand, there is often an element of uncertainty, and full reassurance cannot be given until every step has been taken to reveal the true state of affairs. *When in doubt, call in expert advice.*

In the case of a cooperative child it may be possible, with head-mirror (or lamp) and Thudichum's speculum, to see and, with small nasal forceps or blunt hooks, to remove the foreign body without general anaesthetic. Local analgesia and decongestion are helpful and may be applied in the form of a small cotton-wool swab wrung out in lidocaine/phenylephrine solution. Extreme care is necessary.

A refractory child should, from the onset, be regarded as a case neces-

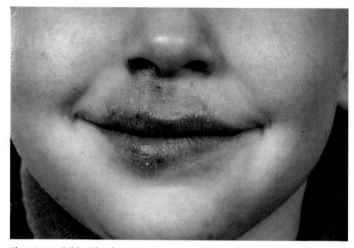

Fig. 18.1 A child with a foreign body in the right nostril.

sitating general anaesthesia. This must be administered by an experienced anaesthetist, and it is usual to employ an endotracheal tube. The surgeon may then remove the foreign body and need have no fear that it will enter the trachea.

Rarely, an adult complaining of nasal obstruction is found to have a large concretion blocking one side of the nose. This is a rhinolith, and consists of many layers of calcium and magnesium salts that have formed around a small central nucleus. The latter often contains a foreign body.

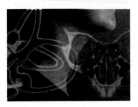

CHAPTER 19

Injuries of the Nose

The nose may be injured in various forms of sport, in personal assaults and in traffic accidents.

Injury to the nose may result in one or a combination of several of the following:

1 epistaxis (see Chapter 20);
2 fractures of the nasal bones;
3 fracture or dislocation of the septum;
4 septal haematoma.

FRACTURE OF THE NASAL BONES (FIG. 19.1)

The fracture is often simple but comminuted. It may be compound, with an open wound in the skin over the nasal bones.

CLINICAL FEATURES

1 Swelling and discoloration of the skin and subcutaneous tissues covering the nasal bones and the vicinity.
2 Tenderness.
3 Mobility of the nose.
4 Deformity. This may or may not be present and is of importance in deciding upon treatment.

TREATMENT

Fractured noses usually bleed and the epistaxis should be controlled first. Lacerations should be cleaned meticulously to avoid tattooing with dirt and sutured carefully with very fine suture material if necessary. X-rays are of doubtful value in nasal fractures and are difficult to interpret. If a previously straight nose is now bent, it must be broken. If it is not bent after an injury, no treatment is necessary. The key to whether treatment is necessary is the presence of deformity, which is more readily appreciated by standing behind the patient and looking down on the nose. If no deformity is present, no manipulation or splinting is required. If deformity is present, decide whether it is bony or cartilaginous. If the nasal bones are displaced, reduction will be necessary.

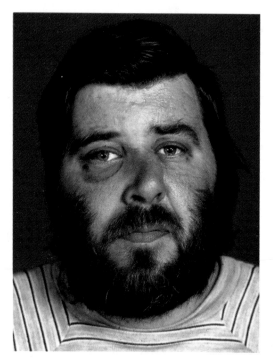

Fig. 19.1 Patient with nasal fracture showing gross displacement of the nasal bones to the left and bruising below the right eye.

When to reduce the fracture

Nasal fractures can be reduced immediately after the injury with little additional discomfort by simple manipulation, but the appropriate medical attendant is rarely present. More often, the patient presents himself to the casualty officer some time later, by which time oedema may obscure the extent of any deformity and preclude manipulation. The oedema will settle over 5–7 days and the patient should be referred to the ENT surgeon within a week of injury. He can then choose the most convenient time to carry out reduction. After 2 weeks, the bone may be so fixed as to render manipulation impossible, and deformity may be permanent. The optimum timing is usually 7–10 days after the injury.

Reduction of fractured nasal bones

The nose should be painted with cocaine paste or sprayed thoroughly with a mixture of lidocaine and phenylephrine to reduce bleeding. Reduction is carried out under general anaesthetic with an endotracheal tube and pharyngeal pack. Anything less than this may be dangerous, because blood can be inhaled. Simple lateral angulation of the nasal bones can often be reduced, with an audible click, by digital pressure on the nose. Depressed nasal fractures will require elevation with Walsham's forceps. If the nasal bones are excessively mobile, splinting with plaster of Paris is necessary.

Nasal fractures are now often reduced in outpatients under local anaesthetic. The nose is cocainized and the external nasal nerve at its exit below the nasal bone is blocked with lignocaine. Nasal bone manipulation can then be carried out with minimal discomfort.

Late treatment of nasal fractures

If a patient with a fractured nose presents months or years after injury, manipulation is clearly not possible, and formal rhinoplasty is necessary. This involves elevation of the skin from the nasal skeleton, mobilization of the nasal bones by lateral saw cuts and realignment. It is a difficult procedure and makes adequate early treatment of nasal fractures all the more important.

Septal dislocation with fracture

Nasal injury may result in deviation of the nasal septum, causing airway obstruction. If no external deformity exists, treatment is by septoplasty or submucous resection (SMR) after a period of weeks or months. Sometimes the septal displacement is accompanied by external nasal deformity that is maintained by the misplaced septum. In such a case, reduction of the nasal bones may be achieved only if the septum is corrected surgically at the same time. Such surgery must be done before the nasal bones have set.

Septal haematoma

Sometimes, soon after a punch on the nose, the victim complains of very severe or complete nasal obstruction. This may be caused by a septal haematoma — the result of haemorrhage between the two sheets of mucoperichondrium covering the septum. It is often (but not always) associated with a fracture of the septum.

The appearance is quite distinctive. Both nasal passages are obliterated by a boggy, pink or dull red swelling replacing the septum.

TREATMENT

Treatment may be expectant in the case of a very small haematoma, but a large one requires incision along the base of the septum, evacuation of the clot, the insertion of a drain, and nasal packing to approximate the septal coverings of muco-perichondrium. Antibiotic cover should be given in an attempt to avert the development of a septal abscess. The patient should be warned that deformity of the nose may ultimately occur (the outcome of necrosis of the cartilage).

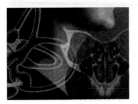

CHAPTER 20

Epistaxis

Epistaxis (nasal bleeding) is a common condition. It may be very severe and life-threatening but in most cases is trivial and easily controlled.

ANATOMY

Bleeding usually arises from the nasal septum, which is supplied by the following vessels:

Anterior ethmoidal artery
Posterior ethmoidal artery } internal carotid artery

Greater palatine
Sphenopalatine artery } external carotid artery
Superior labial artery

These vessels form a rich plexus on the anterior part of the septum — Little's area. Bleeding is less common from the lateral nasal wall, but is more difficult to control.

AETIOLOGY

In many cases of epistaxis, no cause is found. However, there are many causes (Table 20.1), two of which are of major importance to the practitioner.

Spontaneous epistaxis

Spontaneous epistaxis is common in children and young adults; it arises from Little's area, it may be precipitated by infection or minor trauma, it is easy to stop, and it tends to recur.

Hypertensive epistaxis

Hypertensive epistaxis affects an older age group. It arises far back or high up in the nose, it is often difficult to stop, and it may recur.

TREATMENT

Treating active epistaxis is a very messy business — cover up your own clothes first.

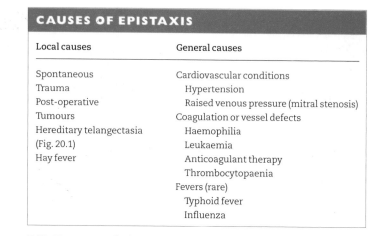

CAUSES OF EPISTAXIS	
Local causes	General causes
Spontaneous	Cardiovascular conditions
Trauma	Hypertension
Post-operative	Raised venous pressure (mitral stenosis)
Tumours	Coagulation or vessel defects
Hereditary telangectasia	Haemophilia
(Fig. 20.1)	Leukaemia
Hay fever	Anticoagulant therapy
	Thrombocytopaenia
	Fevers (rare)
	Typhoid fever
	Influenza

Table 20.1 Causes of epistaxis.

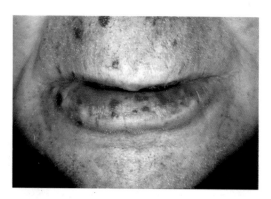

Fig. 20.1 The lesions of hereditary telangectasia.

Bleeding from Little's area

1   Direct digital pressure on the lower nose compresses the vessel on the septum and will arrest the bleeding. Pressure at the root of the nose over the nasal bones is useless.

2   Paint the nasal septum with cocaine paste or apply a plug of cotton wool soaked in lidocaine and phenylephrine and leave for 5–10 min.

3   Cauterize the bleeding point. This can be done with silver nitrate crystals fused to a wire, or with a proprietary silver nitrate stick.

4   Electric cautery or diathermy can be performed—under local anaesthetic in cooperative adults and under general anaesthetic in children. It is more effective than chemicals when there is active bleeding.

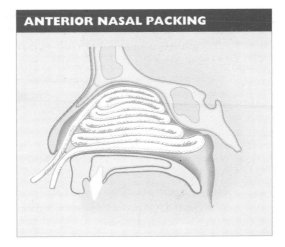

ANTERIOR NASAL PACKING

Fig. 20.2 Anterior nasal packing.

Bleeding from an unidentified site

1   Apply direct digital pressure to the nose for 10 minutes. The patient should sit leaning forward to allow the blood to trickle, and should breathe through the mouth. Swallowing, which may dislodge a clot, is forbidden.

2   Examine the nose with good lighting and spray with lidocaine and phenylephrine solution if available. If a bleeding site is visible, cauterize it with silver nitrate or bipolar diathermy.

3   Nasal packing. If simple measures fail to control the bleeding, the nose will need to be packed using 1-inch ribbon gauze (Fig. 20.2). The pack can be impregnated with BIPP (bismuth and iodoform paste). The pack is introduced along the floor of the nose and built up in loops towards the roof, applying even pressure to the nasal mucosa.

Alternatively, an inflatable pack such as a Brighton balloon can be introduced. It is easier to put in but may not be as effective.

A further and easier option is to use self-expanding packs such as Merocel which enlarge in the presence of moisture.

4   Post-nasal packing may be necessary if the bleeding is from far back — this is best left to the experts as it is not easy.

Elderly patients with epistaxis severe enough to need packing should normally be admitted to hospital. With bed rest and sedation, most cases will settle. The blood pressure should be monitored and the haemoglobin level checked. Coexistent hypertension may need to be controlled.

SURGICAL TREATMENT

Surgical treatment is rarely necessary.

1   Submucous resection (SMR) if the bleeding is from behind a septal spur or if deviation prevents packing.

2   Ligation of the ethmoidal arteries via the medial orbit.

3   Ligation of the external carotid artery (an easy procedure) or of the sphenopalatine artery by nasal endoscopic surgery (a more difficult procedure).

4   Angiography and vessel embolization may be necessary in rare cases of persistent bleeding.

NB. Epistaxis may be severe and may kill the patient. Circulatory resuscitation may be necessary before trying to arrest the bleeding. Do not delay in setting up an intravenous infusion if the patient has circulatory collapse, and at the same time send blood for cross-matching.

CHAPTER 21

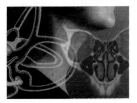

The Nasal Septum

SEPTAL DEVIATION

The nasal septum is rarely midline but marked degrees of deviation will cause nasal airway obstruction. In most cases it can be corrected by surgery, with excellent results.

AETIOLOGY

Most cases of deviated nasal septum (DNS) result from trauma, either recent or long forgotten, perhaps during birth. Buckling in children may become more pronounced as the septum grows.

SYMPTOMS

1 Nasal obstruction — may be unilateral or bilateral.
2 Recurrent sinus infection due to impairment of sinus ventilation by the displaced septum. Alternatively, the middle turbinate on the concave side of the septum may hypertrophy and interfere with sinus ventilation.
3 Recurrent serous otitis media. It has been shown that DNS may impair the ability to equalize middle-ear pressure, especially in divers.

SIGNS

Two main deformities occur and may coexist. First, the caudal end of the septum may be dislocated laterally from the columella, narrowing one nostril, while the septal cartilage lies obliquely in the nose causing narrowing of the opposite side (Fig. 21.1). Second, the septum may be convex to one side, often associated with inferior dislocation of the cartilage from the maxillary crest to cause a visible spur.

The changes present in the nasal septum are easily seen on examination of the nose with a nasal speculum. It is helpful to try to recognize the anatomical deformation that has occurred (Fig. 21.2).

TREATMENT

If symptoms are minimal and only a minor degree of deviation is present, no treatment is necessary other than treatment of coexisting conditions, such as nasal allergy.

DEVIATION OF NASAL SEPTUM

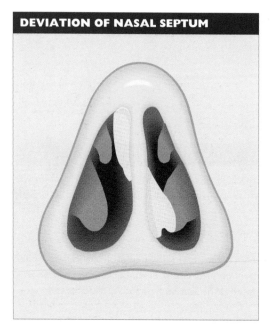

Fig. 21.1 'S'-shaped deviation of the nasal septum with hypertrophy of the right middle turbinate.

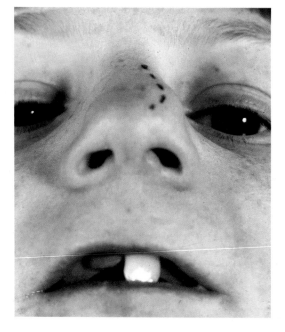

Fig. 21.2 The dorsal line of the nasal septum has been marked and is displaced to the left, causing external nasal deformity in addition to nasal obstruction.

SUBMUCOUS RESECTION OF THE SEPTUM

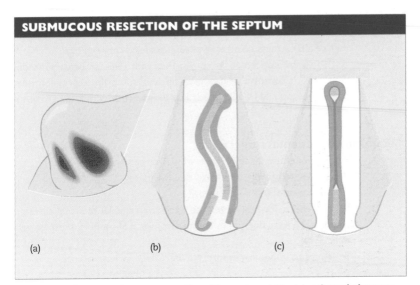

(a)   (b)   (c)

Fig. 21.3 Submucous resection of the septum. (a) Incision through the muco-perichondrium. (b) Elevation of muco-perichondrial flaps on either side of the septal skeleton. (c) The displaced cartilage and bone has been resected, allowing the septum to resume a midline position.

    Where more severe symptoms are present, correction of the septal deformity is justified (though never essential).

Submucous resection (SMR)

SMR (Fig. 21.3) is the operation of choice for mid-septal deformity when the caudal septum is in a normal position. It is to be avoided in children, because interference with nasal growth will occur, leading, in turn, to collapse of the nasal dorsum.

    Under local or general anaesthetic, an incision is made 1 cm back from the front edge of the cartilage through the muco-perichondrium, which is elevated from the cartilage. The incision is then deepened through the cartilage and the muco-perichondrium on the other side is elevated.

    Deflected cartilage and bone are removed with punch forceps and the two mucosal flaps are allowed to fall back into the midline.

    The nose is packed gently for 24 h to maintain apposition of the flaps and the patient may go home after 2 days.

Septoplasty

Septoplasty is the operation of choice (i) in children, (ii) when combined with rhinoplasty, and (iii) when there is dislocation of the caudal end of the septal cartilage. The essential features of septoplasty are a minimum of cartilage removal and careful repositioning of the septal skeleton in the midline after straightening or removing spurs and convexities.

It may be performed in conjunction with mid- or posterior-septal resection. It avoids the drooping tip and supra-tip depression seen sometimes after SMR and causes less interference with facial growth in children.

Complications of septal surgery

1   Post-operative haemorrhage, which may be severe.
2   Septal haematoma, which may require drainage.
3   Septal perforation—see below.
4   External deformity—owing to excessive removal of septal cartilage, allowing the nasal dorsum to collapse from lack of support. It can be very difficult to correct.
5   Anosmia—fortunately rare, but untreatable when it occurs.

SEPTAL PERFORATION

AETIOLOGY

Perforation of the nasal septum is most common in its anterior cartilaginous part and may result from the following conditions:

1   postoperative (particularly SMR);
2   nose-picking (ulceration occurs first, perforation later);
3   trauma;
4   Wegener's granuloma;
5   inhalation of fumes of chrome salts;
6   cocaine addiction;
7   rodent ulcer (basal cell carcinoma);
8   lupus;
9   syphilis (the gumma affects the entire septum and nasal bones, with resulting deformity).

SYMPTOMS

Symptoms consist of epistaxis and crusting, which may cause considerable obstruction. Occasionally, whistling on inspiration or expiration is present. Frequently, the subject is symptom-free.

SIGNS

A perforation is readily seen and often has unhealthy edges covered with large crusts.

INVESTIGATION

In any case where the cause is not clear, the following should be carried out:

1   full blood count and ESR to exclude Wegener's granuloma;
2   urinalysis, especially for haematuria;
3   chest X-ray;
4   serology for syphilis;
5   if doubt remains, a biopsy from the edge of the perforation is taken.

TREATMENT

Septal perforations are almost impossible to repair. If whistling is a problem, enlargement of the perforation relieves the patient's embarrassment.

Nasal douching with saline or bicarbonate solution reduces crusting around the edge of the defect, and antiseptic cream will control infection.

If crusting and bleeding remain a problem, the perforation can be closed using a silastic double-flanged button.

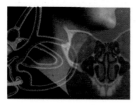

CHAPTER 22

Miscellaneous
Nasal Infections

Acute coryza

The common cold is the result of viral infection but secondary bacterial infection may supervene. Its course is self-limiting and no treatment is required other than an antipyretic, such as aspirin. The prolonged use of vasoconstrictor nose drops should be discouraged, owing to their harmful effect on nasal mucosa (rhinitis medicamentosa).

Nasal vestibulitis

Both children and adults may be carriers of pyogenic staphylococci, which can produce infection of the skin of the nasal vestibule. The site becomes sore and fissured and crusting will occur. Treatment, which needs to be prolonged, consists of topical antibiotic/antiseptic ointment and systemic flucloxacillin. Always take a swab for culture and sensitivity.

Furunculosis

Abscess in a hair follicle is rare but must be treated seriously as it can lead to cavernous sinus thrombosis. The tip of the nose becomes red, tense and painful. Systemic antibiotics should be given without delay, preferably by injection. Drainage may be necessary but should be deferred until the patient has had adequate antibiotic treatment for 24 h. In recurrent cases, diabetes must be excluded.

Chronic purulent rhinitis

Chronic purulent nasal discharge may occur, especially in children. The discharge is thick, mucoid and incessant and often resistant to treatment. In such cases, a nasal swab may show the presence of *Haemophilus influenzae*, which should be treated with a prolonged course of antibiotics (amoxycillin, cotrimoxazole).

It is necessary to exclude immunological deficiency, cystic fibrosis and ciliary abnormality in such cases of chronic rhinitis, as well as more obvious causes, such as enlarged adenoids, foreign body or allergic rhinitis.

Atrophic rhinitis (ozaena)

Fortunately now uncommon in Western society, this disease is still seen occasionally. The nasal mucosa undergoes squamous metaplasia followed by atrophy, and the nose becomes filled with evil-smelling crusts, the stench of which is detectable even at a considerable distance. Such a patient will be ostracized and children will be abused by their peers.

The aetiology of atrophic rhinitis is unknown. Various forms of treatment have been tried. In the early stages, meticulous attention to sinusitis and nasal hygiene may be helpful. In the more established case, the use of 50% glucose in glycerine as nasal drops seems to reduce the smell and crusting.

Various surgical measures have been devised, the most reliable of which is closure of the nostrils, using a circumferential flap of vestibular skin. After a prolonged period of closure, recovery of the nasal mucosa may occur and the nose can be reopened (Young's operation).

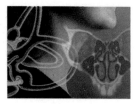

CHAPTER 23

Acute and Chronic Sinusitis

MAXILLARY SINUSITIS

Anatomy and physiology

The maxillary antrum is pyramidal and has a capacity in the adult of approximately 15 mL. Above it lies the orbit. Behind it is the pterygo-palatine fossa containing the maxillary artery. Inferiorly hard palate forms the floor and lies close to the roots of the second premolar and the first two molar teeth. Medially the antrum is separated from the nose by the lateral nasal wall made up of the middle and inferior turbinate bones, each with a corresponding recess or meatus below it (Fig. 23.1).

The ethmoidal sinuses form a honey-comb of air cells between the lamina papyracea of the orbit and the upper part of the nose. An upward extension forms the fronto-nasal duct draining the frontal sinus.

The openings of the sinuses under the middle turbinate form the ostio-meatal complex and it is now recognized that abnormality of this area leads to failure of sinus drainage and thence to sinusitis.

Abnormalities may be structural, as with a large aerated cell blocking the ostial openings, or may be functional such as oedema, allergy or polyp formation. The key to treatment of sinusitis lies in recognition of the abnormality and its correction by surgery or medication.

ACUTE INFECTION

AETIOLOGY

Most cases of acute sinusitis are secondary to:

1 common cold;
2 influenza;
3 measles, whooping cough, etc.

In about 10% of cases the infection is dental in origin, as in:

1 apical abscess;
2 dental extraction.

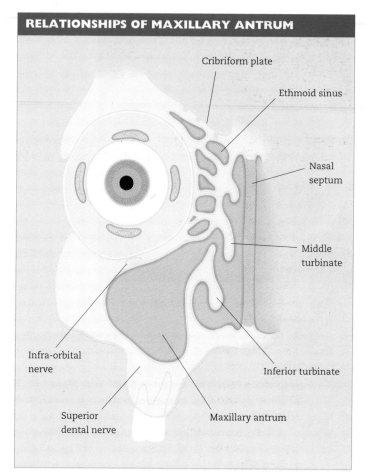

RELATIONSHIPS OF MAXILLARY ANTRUM

Cribriform plate

Ethmoid sinus

Nasal septum

Middle turbinate

Infra-orbital nerve

Inferior turbinate

Superior dental nerve

Maxillary antrum

Fig. 23.1 The anatomical relationships of the maxillary antrum.

Occasionally, infection follows the entry of infected material, as in:
1 diving—water is forced through the ostium, into the sinus;
2 fractures;
3 gunshot wounds.

SYMPTOMS

1 The patient usually has an upper respiratory tract infection, or gives a history of dental infection or recent extraction.
2 Pain over the maxillary antrum, often referred to the supra-orbital

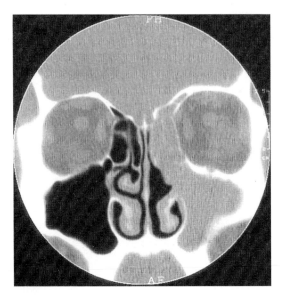

Fig. 23.2 Coronal CT scan showing left-sided ethmoidal and maxillary sinusitis.

region. The pain is usually throbbing and is aggravated by bending, coughing or walking.

3   Nasal obstruction—may be unilateral if unilateral sinusitis is present.

PATHOLOGY

The causative organisms are usually *streptococcus pneumoniae*, *Haemophilus influenzae* or *Staphylococcus pyogenes*. In dental infections, anaerobes may be present.

The mucous membrane of the sinuses becomes inflamed and oedematous and pus forms. If the ostia are obstructed by oedema, the antrum becomes filled with pus under pressure—empyema of the antrum.

SIGNS

I   Pyrexia is usually present.
2   Tenderness over the antrum and on percussion of the upper teeth.
3   Mucopus in the nose or in the nasopharynx.
4   There may be dental caries or an oro-antral fistula.
5   X-ray shows opacity or a fluid level in the antrum (Fig. 23.2).

Three important rules

I   Swelling of the cheek is very rare in maxillary sinusitis.
2   Swelling of the cheek is most commonly of dental origin.
3   Swelling of the cheek as a result of antral disease usually indicates carcinoma of the maxillary antrum.

TREATMENT

1 The patient should be off work and should rest.

2 An appropriate antibiotic should be started after taking a nasal swab. Amoxycillin (to take account of *Haemophilus*) is a good first-time treatment.

3 Vasoconstrictor nose drops, such as 1% ephedrine or 0.05% oxymetazoline, will aid drainage of the sinus.

4 Analgesics.

In most cases, resolution of acute maxillary sinusitis will occur, but on occasion antral wash-out will be necessary to drain pus.

Chronic sinusitis

Most cases of acute sinusitis resolve but some progress to chronicity. This is particularly likely to happen if there is an abnormality of the anatomy, allergy, polyps or immune deficit.

SYMPTOMS

1 Patients with chronic maxillary sinusitis usually have very few symptoms.

2 There is usually nasal obstruction and anosmia.

3 There is usually nasal or postnasal discharge of mucopus.

4 Cacosmia may occur in infections of dental origin.

SIGNS

1 Mucopus in the middle meatus under the middle turbinate.

2 Nasal mucosa congested.

3 Imaging shows fluid level or opacity, or mucosal thickening within the sinus.

TREATMENT

Medical

A further course of treatment with antibiotics, vasoconstrictor nose drops and steam inhalations is worthwhile, as it may produce resolution.

Functional endoscopic surgery

Developments in endoscopic instruments allow inspection of the sinus ostia and interior of the antrum. Ostial enlargement and removal of polyps and cysts can be performed. The ostio-meatal complex under the middle turbinate is opened up and allows more physiological drainage of the antrum than inferior meatal antrostomy.

ACUTE FRONTAL SINUSITIS

This may occur as an isolated condition but more usually forms part of more widespread sinus infection.

TREATMENT

1 Bed rest.
2 Antibiotics—amoxycillin plus metronidazole will cover the most likely organisms.
3 Nasal decongestants—0.5% ephedrine or 0.05% oxymetazoline.
4 Analgesics.
5 In severe cases where, despite intensive therapy, there is increasing oedema and redness of the eyelid, the frontal sinus must be drained. An incision is made below the medial one-third of the eyebrow and a trephine opening made into the sinus. A drainage tube is inserted, through which the sinus can be irrigated.

CLINICAL FEATURES OF FRONTAL SINUSITIS

The symptoms and signs are similar to those of acute maxillary sinusitis, with the following additional features:
1 the pain is mainly supra-orbital;
2 the pain may be periodic (present in the morning; very severe at midday; subsides during the afternoon);
3 acute tenderness is elicited by upward pressure under the floor of the sinus or by percussion of its anterior wall;
4 oedema of the upper eyelid may be present;
5 X-rays show opacity or fluid level in frontal sinus, and usually opacity of ethmoids and maxillary sinus.

Box 23.1 Clinical features of frontal sinusitis.

COMPLICATIONS (Fig. 23.3)

1 Orbital complication (cellulitis or abscess) are characterized by diplopia, marked oedema of the eyelids, chemosis of the conjunctiva and sometimes proptosis. Resolution usually follows intensive antibiotic therapy and local drainage but surgical drainage is required urgently if there is any change in vision. Loss of colour discrimination is an early sign of impending visual loss.
2 Meningitis, extradural and subdural abscesses may occur and should be treated as neurosurgical emergencies.

COMPLICATIONS OF FRONTAL SINUSITIS

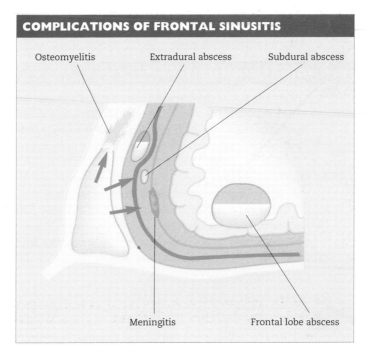

Osteomyelitis   Extradural abscess   Subdural abscess

Meningitis   Frontal lobe abscess

Fig. 23.3 Complications of frontal sinusitis.

3 Cerebral abscess (frontal lobe) deserves special mention in view of the insidious nature of its development. Any patient who has a history of recent frontal sinus infection and complains of headaches, is apathetic or exhibits any abnormality of behaviour should be suspected of harbouring a frontal lobe abscess.

4 Osteomyelitis of the frontal bone is characterized by persistent headache and oedema of the scalp in the vicinity of the frontal sinus. X-ray signs are late, and by the time they become apparent osteomyelitis is well established. Sequestration may occur, and intensive antibiotic therapy combined with removal of diseased bone is necessary.

5 Cavernous sinus thrombosis is very rare. Proptosis, chemosis and ophthalmoplegia characterize this dangerous complication.

Recurrent and chronic infection

Recurring acute or persisting chronic infection may become established. Treatment is by antibiotics and topical steroids. If surgery is necessary, it is now usual to establish drainage by endoscopic surgery of the ostio-meatal area under the middle turbinate. Only rarely is external fronto-ethmoidectomy necessary.

ETHMOIDAL SINUSITIS

Acute infection of the ethmoidal complex usually follows a coryzal cold. The area becomes swollen and inflamed. There may be gross oedema of the eyelids and rupture into the orbit may occur. Pressure on the optic nerve endangers the sight in the affected eye (see above under frontal sinusitis).

TREATMENT

In the early stages antibiotics should prove curative but if abscess formation is suspected, it may be confirmed by CT or MR scan. Either external drainage by external ethmoidectomy, or intranasal drainage by endoscopic surgery is performed to drain pus and relieve pressure on the orbit.

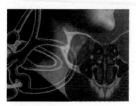

CHAPTER 24

Tumours of the Nose, Sinuses and Nasopharynx

CARCINOMA OF THE MAXILLARY ANTRUM

CLINICAL FEATURES

Early

Carcinoma of the maxillary antrum is seldom diagnosed until it has spread to surrounding structures. In its earliest stages it will give rise to no symptoms, but blood-stained nasal discharge and increasing unilateral nasal obstruction should raise suspicion.

Late

1. Swelling of the cheek.
2. Swelling or ulceration of the bucco-alveolar sulcus or palate.
3. Epiphora, owing to involvement of the nasal lacrimal duct.
4. Proptosis and diplopia, owing to involvement of the floor of the orbit.
5. Pain — commonly in the distribution of the second division of the fifth nerve, but may be referred via other branches to the ear, head or mandible.

Spread

Local extension beyond the bony confines of the antrum is not long delayed and may involve the following: cheek, buccal sulcus, palate, nasal cavity and naso-lacrimal duct, infra-orbital nerve, orbit and pterygopalatine fossa.

Lymphatic spread is to the submandibular and deep cervical nodes and occurs late.

Distant metastases are rare.

INVESTIGATIONS

1. CT scanning is invaluable to assess the extent of invasion and bone erosion (Fig. 24.1).
2. MR scanning will show the extent of soft tissue mass.
3. Biopsy — often the tumour will have spread into the nasal cavity, whence a biopsy is easily obtained. If the tumour is still within the confines of the antrum, a specimen is obtained via the antronasal wall.

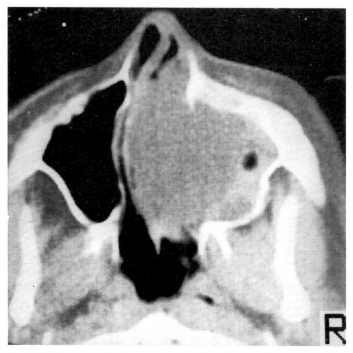

Fig. 24.1 CT scan showing large carcinoma of the right maxillary antrum with extension into the right nasal cavity.

TREATMENT

A combination of surgery and radiotherapy offers the best chance of cure. First, maxillectomy (with exenteration of the orbit if involved) is carried out. This results in fenestration of the hard palate, for which a modified upper denture with an obturator is provided. The fenestration allows drainage and access for inspection of the antral cavity. Following maxillectomy, a radical course of radiotherapy is given.

This aggressive combination of treatments is justified by the poor prognosis of the disease if not treated adequately from the outset.

PROGNOSIS

Even with radical treatment, carcinoma of the antrum has a poor prognosis, with only about 30% of patients surviving to 5 years.

CARCINOMA OF THE ETHMOID SINUSES

The clinical features are similar to those of maxillary carcinoma, but invasion of the orbit and facial skin below the inner canthus is early. Treatment is by radical surgery and radiotherapy.

MALIGNANT DISEASE OF THE NASOPHARYNX

Rare in Europe but relatively common in southern China, malignant disease of the nasopharynx often causes difficulty in diagnosis because of the absence of local symptoms.

PATHOLOGY

Virtually all malignant tumours of the nasopharynx are squamous cell carcinoma, but rarely lymphoma or adenoid cystic carcinoma may occur. Cancer of the nasopharynx spreads locally to invade the skull base and Eustachian tube and metastasizes early to the upper deep cervical lymph nodes. The Epstein–Barr virus may play a role in the aetiology of nasopharyngeal malignancy.

CLINICAL FEATURES

Local. Nasal obstruction, blood-stained nasal discharge — usually a late development.

Otological. Unilateral serous otitis media will result from Eustachian tube obstruction.

Neurological. Invasion of the skull base causes paralysis of various cranial nerves, especially nerves V, VI, IX, X and XII.

Cervical. Spread to the upper deep cervical nodes occurs early and may be bilateral. Such a node is typically wedged between the mastoid process and angle of the jaw.

It is inexcusable, and dangerous, to biopsy such nodes until the nasopharynx has been examined and biopsied. The combination of unilateral deafness, enlarged cervical nodes and cranial nerve palsies proclaims the diagnosis of nasopharyngeal cancer loud and clear.

TREATMENT

Treatment of nasopharyngeal cancer is by radiotherapy following confirmatory biopsy. Once the primary site has been controlled, radical neck dissection is carried out if there were involved nodes at diagnosis or if any subsequently develop. The prognosis is poor, but the earlier the diagnosis is made, the better the outlook.

OTHER TUMOURS OF THE NASAL REGION

Osteomata

Osteomata occur in the frontal and ethmoidal sinuses. They are slow-growing and cause few symptoms but may eventually call for surgical removal.

Nasopharyngeal angiofibroma

Nasopharyngeal angiofibroma is a rare tumour of adolescent boys. It presents as epistaxis and nasal obstruction and is usually easily visible by posterior rhinoscopy. Being highly vascular, the tumour is locally destructive and extends into the surrounding structures. Diagnosis is confirmed by angiography and treatment is by surgical removal.

Malignant granuloma

Though not truly neoplastic, malignant granuloma is a sinister condition characterized by progressive ulceration of the nose and neighbouring structures. There are two main varieties: the Stewart type, in which the lesion is limited to the skull and is characterized by a pleomorphic histiocytic infiltration and which is a form of lymphoma; and the Wegener type, in which the kidneys, lungs and other tissues may show periarteritis, the local nasal lesion containing multinucleated giant cells. It is probable that Wegener's granuloma is an auto-immune disease. Radiotherapy, steroids and cytotoxic agents are used in its treatment and occasionally are successful.

Malignant melanoma

Malignant melanoma is fortunately rare in the nose and sinuses. Treatment is by radical surgery but the prognosis is extremely poor.

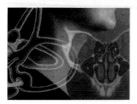

CHAPTER 25

Allergic Rhinitis, Vasomotor Rhinitis and Nasal Polyps

Hypersensitivity of the nasal and sinus mucosa may be allergic or nonallergic in aetiology. Allergic rhinitis is mediated by reaginic antibody (IgE). Non-allergic vasomotor rhinitis does not involve the type I allergic response. It may be subdivided into the eosinophilic type, in which there are abundant eosinophils in the nasal secretion, and the non-eosinophilic type, which is probably secondary to autonomic dysfunction.

ALLERGIC RHINITIS

Following exposure to a particular allergen, the susceptible individual produces reaginic antibody (IgE), which becomes bound to the surface of a mast cell (Fig. 25.1). Such cells abound in nasal mucosa and when fixed to IgE molecules are said to be sensitized. Further exposure to the specific allergen causes its binding to the IgE of the sensitized mast cell, degranulation of the cell and release of histamine, slow-reacting substance and vasoactive peptides (Fig. 25.2). These substances cause vasodilation, increased capillary permeability and smooth-muscle contraction — the features of allergic airways disease.

The atopic syndrome

The atopic syndrome is a hereditary disorder of variable penetrance. Subjects are particularly susceptible to the development of IgE-mediated allergic reactions manifested by:

1 infantile eczema;
2 allergic asthma;
3 nasal and conjunctival allergy.

Allergens

The allergens responsible for nasal allergy are inhaled and may be:

1 seasonal, e.g. mould spores in autumn, tree and grass pollen in spring;
2 perennial, e.g. animal dander (especially cats), house dust mite (Fig. 25.3).

SYMPTOMS

1 Watery rhinorrhoea.

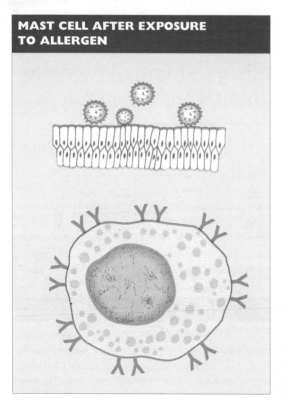

MAST CELL AFTER EXPOSURE TO ALLERGEN

Fig. 25.1 A mast cell showing intracellular granules and antibodies attached to the cell wall.

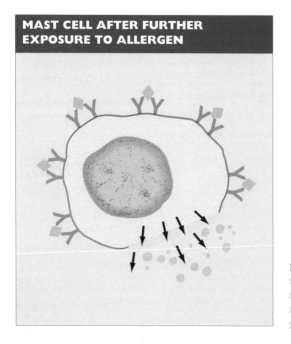

MAST CELL AFTER FURTHER EXPOSURE TO ALLERGEN

Fig. 25.2 Further exposure to antigen has resulted in rupture of the cell wall and release of the mast cell granules.

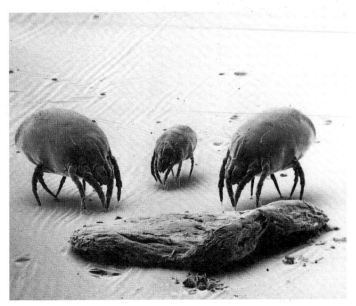

Fig. 25.3 Scanning electron microscopy of house dust mites and a human squame. (Crown copyright reproduced by kind permission of Dr DA Griffiths, Head of Storage Pests Department, Slough Laboratory, London Road, Slough.)

2   Sneezing attacks — often violent and prolonged.
3   Nasal obstruction.
4   Conjunctival irritation and lacrimation.
In taking a history, it is important to relate the onset of the symptoms to exposure to the suspected allergen.

SIGNS

1   The nasal mucosa is oedematous and usually pale or violet in colour.
2   There is excessive clear mucus within the nose, and this usually contains an increased number of eosinophils.
3   Children may develop a transverse nasal skin crease from rubbing the nose — the allergic salute.

INVESTIGATIONS

1   The importance of a history of symptoms related to allergen exposure cannot be overemphasized.
2   Skin testing interpreted in relation to the history is valuable. The skin of the forearm is pricked with a needle through a dilute solution of

the relevant allergen; a positive response is a central weal with surrounding erythema.

3 RAST (radio-allergo sorbent test) measures allergen-specific IgE and has the advantage of being performed on a blood sample. It is especially useful in children for whom skin tests are unsuitable.

4 A high total IgE level is a useful indication of the presence of atopy.

TREATMENT

1 Avoidance of contact with the allergen may be possible, especially in the case of domestic pets.

2 Antihistamines are useful in acute episodes but tolerance develops. The latest generation of antihistamines (H_1 receptor antagonists) do not produce drowsiness.

3 Vasoconstrictor nasal drops provide temporary relief but are not advisable, as prolonged use leads to chronic rhinitis medicamentosa.

4 Sodium cromoglycate (Rynacrom) applied to the nose 4–6 times daily as prophylaxis is particularly suitable for children.

5 Topically applied steroid preparations (beclomethasone, flunisolide) are probably the most effective treatment of nasal allergy. Systemic effects of steroid therapy are absent but such treatment is not advisable in young children.

6 Desensitization by administration of increasing dosages of allergen is no longer widely practised, as it is of little benefit in most cases and carries the risk of anaphylaxis.

7 If gross hypertrophy of the nasal mucosa has occurred, surgical reduction by diathermy or laser may be beneficial.

NON-ALLERGIC VASOMOTOR RHINITIS

Eosinophilic vasomotor rhinitis

Eosinophilic vasomotor rhinitis is associated with the formation of nasal polyps, aspirin sensitivity and asthma. The symptoms are similar to allergic rhinitis with watery rhinorrhoea and sneezing, but the type I allergic response is not involved. There may, however, be increased nasal sensitivity to irritants such as perfume and tobacco smoke. Although a blood count may not always show a raised eosinophil count, such cells will be present in nasal secretions.

TREATMENT

Treatment is by topical nasal steroid (e.g. beclomethasone) or systemic

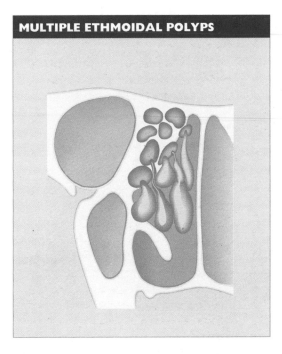

MULTIPLE ETHMOIDAL POLYPS

Fig. 25.4 Multiple
ethmoidal polyps.

antihistamine and the response is usually good. Topical ipratropium may
control the rhinorrhea.

Nasal polyps

Nasal polyps occur in nonallergic eosinophilic rhinitis rather than in allergic
rhinitis. They cause nasal obstruction, sometimes with a ball-valve effect,
nasal discharge, and are usually bilateral. They have a tendency to recur.

Diagnosis is made by examination of the nose. Polyps are yellowish-grey
or pink, smooth and moist (Fig. 25.4). They are pedunculated and move on
probing. It is a common error to see the inferior turbinate and mistake it for
a polyp—do not be caught out.

Nasal polyps do not occur in children except in the presence of cystic
fibrosis. An apparent polyp in a baby is probably a nasal glioma or a nasal
encephalocoele.

Histologically, nasal polyps consist of a loose oedematous stroma
infiltrated by inflammatory lymphocytes and eosinophils and covered by
respiratory epithlium.

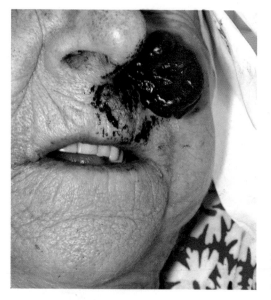

Fig. 25.5 A nasal polyp which has prolapsed out of the nose.

TREATMENT

1 Nasal polyps may shrink with topical steroid therapy but will not usually disappear.

2 Nasal polypectomy is performed under local or general anaesthetic, the polyps being removed with grasping forceps or by a powered microdebrider.

3 Endoscopic ethmoidectomy may be required for recalcitrant cases

4 Short courses of steroids are useful in severe cases.

Antrochoanal polyps

An antrochoanal polyp is usually solitary, arising within the maxillary antrum, extruding through the ostium and presenting as a smooth swelling in the nasopharynx (Fig. 25.5). Such a polyp may extend below the soft palate and be several centimetres in length. Treatment consists of avulsion from within the nose and delivering the polyp, usually per-orally.

Non-eosinophilic vasomotor rhinitis

Non-eosinophilic vasomotor rhinitis (Fig. 25.6) is less common than its eosinophilic counterpart and is thought to be due to autonomic disturbance of vasomotor tone, with excessive parasympathetic activity.

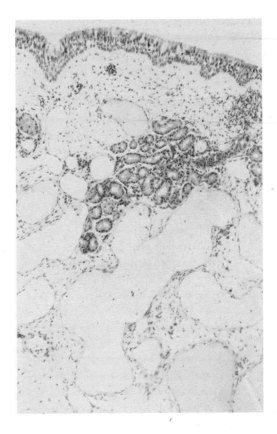

Fig. 25.6 View of nasal turbinate mucosa showing the many blood vessels within the substance. (Slide courtesy of Dr Roger Start.)

AETIOLOGY

In most cases no specific cause is found but certain conditions may be relevant.

1 Drug treatment: certain antihypertensive drugs, particularly ganglion blockers; contraceptive pills; vasodilator drugs.

2 Hormonal disturbance: pregnancy; menopause; hypothyroidism.

3 Congestive cardiac failure.

4 Anxiety state.

5 Occupational irritants, e.g. ammonia, sulphur dioxide.

6 Smoking.

SYMPTOMS

1 Watery rhinorrhoea.

2 Nasal obstruction—varies from side to side and is worse on lying down, especially in the undermost nostril.

3 Sneezing attacks.

Symptoms are often precipitated by change of temperature, bright sunlight, irritants (e.g. tobacco smoke) or alcohol ingestion.

SIGNS

1   There may be none. Usually the nasal mucosa is dusky and congested, the engorgement of the inferior turbinates leading to the nasal obstruction.
2   There may be excessive secretions in the nose.
3   The symptoms are often more severe than examination of the nose would suggest.

TREATMENT

1   Often no treatment is required because the symptoms are minor and no significant abnormality is found on examination.
2   Exercise, by increasing sympathetic tone, often provides relief.
3   Sympathomimetic drugs, e.g. 15 mg pseudoephedrine t.d.s., are often helpful but tolerance occurs rapidly (tachyphylaxis).
4   The watery rhinorrhoea may respond to topical nasal ipratropium spray, but this has no effect on nasal blockage.
5   If hypertrophy of the nasal mucosa has occurred, surgical reduction by diathermy, cryosurgery or amputation is of value.
6   Vasoconstrictor nose drops, such as oxymetazoline, should be condemned. Such strictures apply also to the use of cromoglycate/vasoconstrictor combinations. Although providing temporary relief, rebound hyperaemia occurs, causing the need for further dosage—a downhill spiral to *rhinitis medicamentosa* will result. Such a habit is hard to break, and the abuse of nasal vasoconstrictor drops is unfortunately widespread and often initiated by medical advisers. There seems to be little justification for the continued availability of this form of therapy.

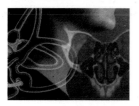

CHAPTER 26

Choanal Atresia

Congenital atresia of the posterior nares is caused by persistence of the bucco-nasal membrane and fortunately is rare. It is often accompanied by other congenital anomalies.

Unilateral atresia

The condition may pass unrecognized until the age of 5–10 years when it becomes apparent that one nostril is occluded and accumulates thick mucus. Testing with a probe and examination by posterior rhinoscopy will confirm the diagnosis (Fig. 26.1).

TREATMENT

Correction of unilateral choanal atresia is perfomed per-nasally, usually with a drill, while observing the choana from the post nasal aspect with a 120° telescope.

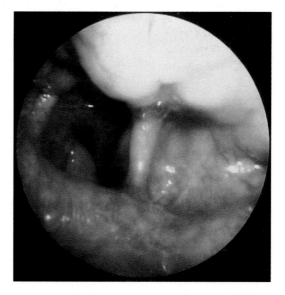

Fig. 26.1 Endoscopic view of unilateral congenital posterior choanal atresia. The atretic plate can be clearly seen, and on the patent side the posterior ends of the inferior and middle turbinates are visible.

Bilateral atresia

This is a life-threatening condition in the newborn infant who is unable to breathe voluntarily through the mouth. It is the only form of airway obstruction that is relieved by crying. It is often associated with other congenital anomalies. Asphyxia will result without immediate first-aid treatment with an oral airway. Such an airway should be fixed in place with sticking plaster, and diagnosis is confirmed by the inability to pass a catheter through the nose into the pharynx. CT scanning shows the atresia clearly.

TREATMENT

Treatment is by surgery, again performed by the transnasal route under endoscopic control.

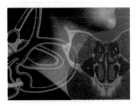

CHAPTER 27

Adenoids

The adenoid mass of lymphoid tissue is situated on the posterior wall of the nasopharynx and occupies much of that cavity in young children. At the age of about 6 or 7 years atrophy commences and, as a rule, by the age of about 15 years little or no adenoid tissue remains. In some children of 1–4 years of age, the adenoids, as a result of repeated upper respiratory infections, undergo hypertrophy with the following ill-effects.

Nasal obstruction

Nasal obstruction becomes established and results in:

1 mouth breathing — the mouth is dry and constantly open;
2 recurrent pharyngeal infections;
3 recurrent chest infections;
4 snoring and disturbed sleep — in severe cases, episodic sleep apnoea may occur.

Eustachian tube

Eustachian tube obstruction predisposes to:

1 recurrent acute otitis media;
2 secretory otitis media with deafness;
3 chronic suppurative otitis media (CSOM).

DIAGNOSIS

The nasal obstruction and mouth breathing are apparent, and the history will confirm the features mentioned above. Diagnosis of enlarged adenoids as the cause of the symptoms is confirmed by mirror examination (Fig. 27.1) or by lateral soft tissue X-ray (Fig. 27.2).

TREATMENT

Adenoidectomy is curative if the case has been selected properly. In children with enlarged adenoids and recurrent aural disease, early adenoidectomy is of supreme importance.

Adenoidectomy is carried out under general anaesthesia with endotracheal intubation. An adenoid curette is swept down the posterior pharyngeal wall, taking care to remove all remnants of lymphoid tissue. Brisk

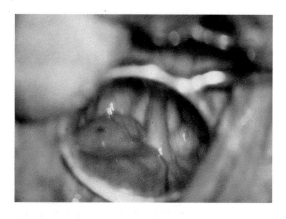

Fig. 27.1 Mirror view of the nasopharynx showing adenoid tissue and the posterior end of the nasal septum. (Viewed under general anaesthetic.)

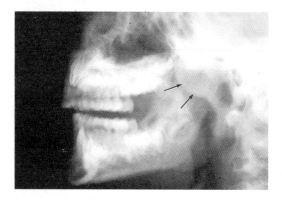

Fig. 27.2 A lateral soft tissue X-ray showing adenoid enlargement.

bleeding usually stops rapidly and the patient remains in the recovery area until fully awake with no persistent bleeding.

COMPLICATIONS

1 Haemorrhage—this usually occurs in the first 24 h. Do not delay in setting up a drip, getting blood cross-matched and returning the child to theatre. *Delay may be fatal.* A postnasal pack is inserted under general anaesthetic after first making sure that there are no tags of adenoid tissue left.

2 Otitis media.

3 Regrowth of residual adenoid tissue.

4 Rhinolalia aperta. Removal of large adenoids in a child with a short soft palate may result in palatal incompetence, with nasal escape during speech. Resolution usually occurs, but if it does not, speech therapy is advisable. Rarely, pharyngoplasty is necessary.

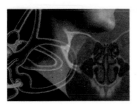

CHAPTER 28

The Tonsils and Oropharynx

Acute tonsillitis

Acute tonsillitis can occur at any age but is most frequent in children under 9 years. Spread is by droplet infection. In infants under 3 years of age with acute tonsillitis, 15% of cases were found to be streptococcal; the remainder were probably viral. In older children, up to 50% of cases are due to *streptococcus pyogenes*. It is commonest in winter and spring.

SYMPTOMS

1   Sore throat and dysphagia. Young children may not complain of sore throat but will refuse to eat.
2   Earache—as a result of referred otalgia.
3   Headache and malaise.

SIGNS

1   Pyrexia is always present and may be high. It may lead to febrile convulsions in susceptible infants.
2   The tonsils are enlarged and hyperaemic and may exude pus from the crypts in follicular tonsillitis.
3   The pharyngeal mucosa is inflamed.
4   Foetor is present.
5   The cervical lymph nodes are enlarged and tender.

DIFFERENTIAL DIAGNOSIS

Infectious mononucleosis

Infectious mononucleosis (glandular fever) usually presents as severe membranous tonsillitis. The node enlargement is marked and malaise is more severe than expected from tonsillitis (Fig. 28.1). Diagnosis is confirmed by lymphocytosis and within a week the monospot test becomes positive.

Scarlet fever

Scarlet fever, now rare, is a streptococcal tonsillitis with added features

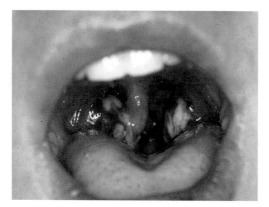

Fig. 28.1 The appearance of the tonsils in glandular fever.

caused by a specific toxin. It is characterized by a punctate erythematous rash, circumoral pallor and a 'strawberry and cream' tongue.

Diphtheria

Diphtheria still occurs on rare occasions in the UK and should be considered in recent travellers to India or the former USSR. It is of insidious onset and characterized by a grey membrane (difficult to remove) on the tonsils, fauces and uvula. Pyrexia is usually low and diagnosis is confirmed by examination and culture of a swab.

Agranulocytosis

Agranulocytosis is manifested by ulceration and membrane formation on the tonsils and oral mucosa. The neutropenia is diagnostic.

HIV

Patients with impaired immunity from HIV infection are particularly at risk of pharyngitis and ulcerative tonsillitis.

TREATMENT OF ACUTE TONSILLITIS

1 Rest—the patient will usually prefer to be in bed.

2 Soluble aspirin or paracetamol held in the mouth and then swallowed eases the discomfort. Remember that aspirin should not be given to children under the age of 12 years because of the risk of Reye's syndrome.

3 Encourage the patient to drink or she/he will easily become dehydrated.

4 Antibiotics in severe cases. Penicillin by injection followed by oral treatment remains the treatment of choice. It is recommended that treatment be continued for 10 days to reduce the risk of reactivation.

There is no place for antiseptic or antibiotic lozenges, which may predispose to monilial infection and are in any case ineffective.

COMPLICATIONS
1 Acute otitis media (the most common complication).
2 Peritonsillar abscess (quinsy).
3 Pulmonary infections (pneumonia, etc.).
4 Acute nephritis IgA nephropathy.
5 Acute rheumatism.

Peritonsillar abscess (quinsy)

CLINICAL FEATURES
A quinsy is a collection of pus forming outside the capsule of the tonsil in close relationship to its upper pole. The abscess occurs as a complication of acute tonsillitis, but is more common in adults than in children.

The patient, already suffering from acute tonsillitis, becomes more ill, has a peak of temperature and develops severe dysphagia with referred otalgia. On examination, a most striking and constant feature is trismus; the buccal mucosa is dirty and foetor is present.

The anatomy of the buccopharyngeal isthmus is distorted by the quinsy, which pushes the adjacent tonsil downwards and medially. The uvula may be so oedematous as to resemble a white grape.

TREATMENT
Systemic penicillin must be given without delay, and in very early cases with 'peritonsillitis' only, abscess formation may be aborted. If much trismus is present and the presence of pus strongly suspected, incision is indicated, for without this, spontaneous rupture may be long-delayed.

If the diagnosis is correct, the patient will spit out pus and some blood, and the relief from former misery is immediate and dramatic.

In children, the drainage of a quinsy should be performed under general anaesthesia; great skill and care are called for to avoid premature rupture of the quinsy before the airway is safeguarded.

Following quinsy, it is conventional to carry out tonsillectomy 6 weeks later. If there has been no previous history of tonsillitis this may not be necessary.

Recurrent acute tonsillitis

Most people will at some time experience acute tonsillitis, but some individuals are subject to recurrent attacks, especially in childhood. Between attacks the patient is usually symptom-free and the tonsils appear healthy. If such attacks are frequent and severe, tonsillectomy is advisable. It is important before arriving at such a decision to be sure that the attacks are truly acute tonsillitis, with the features listed earlier. If there is doubt, it is helpful to ask the patient (or the parents) to document the attacks over a period of several months. If there are contraindications to operation, e.g. a bleeding disorder, long-term prophylaxis with oral penicillin may reduce the frequency and severity of attacks.

Tonsillar enlargement

As a general rule, the size of the tonsils is immaterial. Many parents are concerned about the size of their offspring's tonsils but can be reassured that no treatment is necessary unless the child is subject to recurring attacks of acute tonsillitis.

There is, however, a small number of children in whom the tonsils and adenoids are enlarged to a degree that makes eating difficult and endangers the airway. Such children are dyspnoeic even at rest, mouth breathe, snore and are prone to episodes of sleep apnoea. Right heart failure may ensue.

A timely operation to remove the tonsils and adenoids from such a child will result in a dramatic improvement in health.

Acute pharyngitis

Acute pharyngitis is exceedingly common, and probably starts as a virus infection. It is often associated with acute nasal infections.

The symptoms consist of dysphagia and malaise and, on examination, the mucosa is found to be hyperaemic.

As a general rule the treatment of acute pharyngitis should consist of regular analgesics, such as aspirin 4–6-hourly. Unhappily, this complaint is frequently treated by course after course of oral antibiotics, often aided and abetted by antibiotic or antiseptic lozenges. As a result, the flora of the mouth and pharynx may be disturbed completely and moniliasis ensues, with the net result that after 6 weeks of treatment little or no progress has been achieved.

Chronic pharyngitis

Chronic pharyngitis produces a persistent though mild soreness of the throat, usually with a complaint of dryness. Examination shows the pharynx to be reddened and there may be enlargement of the lymphoid nodules on the posterior pharyngeal wall — granular pharyngitis. There may also be present lateral bands of lymphoid tissue alongside the posterior faucial pillars.

Predisposing factors that should be looked for are:

1   smoking or excessive indulgence in spirit drinking;
2   mouth breathing as a result of nasal obstruction;
3   chronic sinusitis;
4   chronic periodontal disease;
5   exposure to harmful fumes, usually industrial;
6   use of antiseptic throat lozenges.

TREATMENT

If any of the causes listed are present, appropriate action will be beneficial. If the lymphoid aggregates on the posterior wall are prominent, treatment by diathermy or cryosurgery may help.

Malignant disease of the tonsil and pharynx

Carcinoma

Carcinoma will present as painful ulceration with induration of the tonsil, fauces or pharyngeal wall. It is often accompanied by referred otalgia and slight bleeding. Lymphatic spread to the upper deep cervical nodes is early. Diagnosis is confirmed by biopsy of the tonsil.

Lymphoma

Lymphoma of the tonsil tends not to ulcerate, but produces painless hypertrophy of the affected tonsil. Tonsillectomy as an excision biopsy is indicated without delay in such a case.

TREATMENT

Treatment of carcinoma is by radical excision usually followed by external irradiation, and of lymphoma by chemotherapy and/or radiotherapy. The prognosis of carcinoma is poor but for lymphoma will depend on its cellular nature, some types having a very good prognosis.

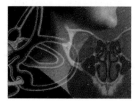

CHAPTER 29

Tonsillectomy

There has been controversy over the removal of tonsils for many decades, with strong opposition and equally strong protagonism. An extreme view defies reason and common sense and to deny tonsillectomy to a child may be to inflict much ill-health and loss of schooling. Equally, the decision to operate must be based on sound evidence that the benefit expected will justify the risk. It is not a trivial operation, and carries a small but real mortality rate.

Indications for operation

1   Recurrent attacks of acute tonsillitis—three or four attacks over a period of a year, or five attacks in 2 years. Always remember that young children are likely to improve spontaneously but such improvement is less likely in adolescents and young adults.

2   Tonsillar and adenoidal hypertrophy causing airway obstruction.

3   Recurrent tonsillitis associated with complications, especially acute or chronic otitis media.

4   Carriers of haemolytic streptococci or diphtheria (a rare indication).

5   Following quinsy.

6   For biopsy in suspected malignancy—this is the only absolute indication for tonsillectomy.

THE OPERATION

1   In the presence of current or recent infection, operation should be postponed.

2   Any suspicion of bleeding disorder must be investigated fully by the haematologist.

3   Any anaemia must be corrected before operation is carried out.

4   The risk of postoperative haemorrhage must be explained to the patient or his parents. It is a brave (or foolhardy) surgeon who embarks on tonsillectomy if blood transfusion is likely to be refused. The time to find out is before the operation.

The operation is carried out under general anaesthetic with endotracheal intubation. The tonsils are removed by careful dissection and haemostasis is obtained by ligating the bleeding vessels. If the adenoids are to be removed at the same operation they are usually dealt with first.

POST-OPERATIVE CARE

The patient will be kept in the recovery area adjacent to the operating theatre until fully conscious. It is vital to ascertain that all bleeding has stopped before being returned to the ward.

Once back on the ward, pulse and blood pressure are checked frequently. The pulse should be taken every half hour for the first four hours and then hourly until discharge. The patient is observed meticulously for any sign of bleeding or airway obstruction.

The care of post-tonsillectomy patients calls for a high degree of vigilance and must never be delegated to inexperienced nurses.

Several hours after operation, most patients are able to take oral fluids but should avoid blackcurrant cordial, which if vomited may look like blood.

After operation, the temperature should be recorded 4-hourly and any rise noted. Pyrexia may be due to local infection, to chest or urinary infections or to otitis media.

Although earache is common after tonsillectomy and is usually referred from the tonsil, do not omit examination of the ears.

The appearance of the tonsillar fossa often gives rise to alarm. Within 12 h it is covered with a yellowish exudate, which persists for 10–14 days. It is quite normal and does not indicate infection. *It is not pus.*

Following tonsillectomy, as normal a diet as possible is to be encouraged. Analgesics, such as soluble paracetamol prior to eating, are helpful. Eating normal food usually produces a reduction in pain afterwards (though not at the time!).

COMPLICATIONS OF TONSILLECTOMY

Reactionary haemorrhage

The major risk from tonsillectomy is that of haemorrhage. Indications of reactionary haemorrhage are:

1 a rising pulse rate, though the blood pressure may remain constant initially;

2 a wet, gurgling sound in the throat on respiration, which clears on swallowing;

3 sudden vomiting of altered or fresh blood, which is often accompanied by circulatory collapse;

4 obvious bleeding from the mouth.

Post-operative bleeding must be stopped urgently and delay may be fatal. Blood must be cross-matched and a drip set up. In a cooperative patient the bleeding may be arrested by the careful removal of clot, followed by pressure from a rolled-up gauze held in forceps. Usually, however, a return to theatre without delay is called for especially in children, when the bleeding point can be identified and ligated. The anaesthetic for such a procedure is hazardous and should not be delegated to a junior anaesthetist.

Secondary haemorrhage

Secondary haemorrhage occurs between the fifth and tenth postoperative days and is due to fibrinolysis aggravated by infection. Such bleeding is rarely profuse but the patient should be readmitted to hospital for observation. Usually the only treatment required is mild sedation and antibiotics, but an intravenous line should always be set up and the blood saved for grouping. It is only rarely necessary to return the patient to the operating theatre to control the bleeding.

Otitis media

Otitis media may occur following tonsillectomy—earache is not referred pain until you are sure the ears are normal.

Infection

Infection may occur in the tonsillar fossae and is marked by pyrexia, foetor and an increase in pain. Secondary haemorrhage is a potential danger and antibiotics should be given.

Pulmonary complications

Pulmonary complications such as pneumonia or lung abscess, are rare and may be caused by inhalation of blood or fragments of tissue.

CHAPTER 30

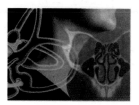

Retropharyngeal Abscess

The condition occurs, as a rule, in infants or young children. Upper respiratory infection causes adenitis in the retropharyngeal lymph nodes, which suppurate. The abscess is limited to one side of the midline by the median raphe of buccopharyngeal fascia, which is firmly attached to the prevertebral fascia (Fig. 30.1).

CLINICAL FEATURES

The infant or child is obviously ill and has a high temperature. Dysphagia is evinced by dribbling, and there may be stridor. The head is often held to one side. Inspection and palpation of the posterior pharyngeal wall reveals a smooth bulge, usually on one side of the midline (Fig. 30.2).

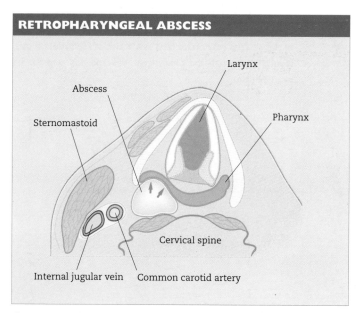

Fig. 30.1 Retropharyngeal abscess. Note the proximity to the larynx and to the great vessels in the parapharyngeal space.

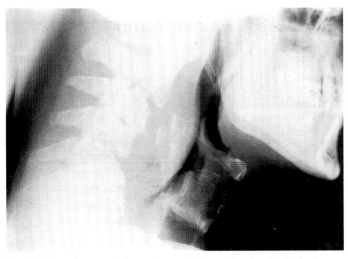

Fig. 30.2 Retropharyngeal abscess in an adult secondary to a foreign body.

TREATMENT

Antibiotics should be given in full doses.

Incision of the abscess should be carried out without delay. General anaesthesia is advisable but requires great skill and gentleness — rupture of the abscess may prove fatal as a result of aspiration of pus. The abscess is incised through the pharyngeal wall and pus sent for bacteriological examination.

CHAPTER 31

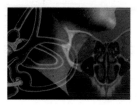

Examination of the Larynx

The visualization of the larynx is obviously of paramount importance in dealing with laryngeal disease, and several methods are available.

INDIRECT LARYNGOSCOPY

This is the most convenient method of examination but it requires instruction and practice.

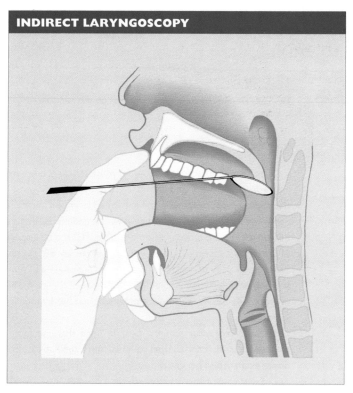

INDIRECT LARYNGOSCOPY

Fig. 31.1 The technique of indirect laryngoscopy.

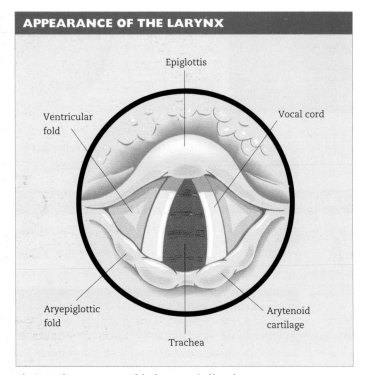

Fig. 31.2 The appearance of the larynx on indirect laryngoscopy.

The patient protrudes his tongue, which is held gently between the examiner's middle finger and thumb (Fig. 31.1). The forefinger is used to hold the upper lip out of the way and a warmed laryngeal mirror is introduced gently but firmly against the soft palate in the midline. By tilting the laryngeal mirror, the various structures shown in Fig. 31.2 can be inspected. Mobility of the cords is assessed by asking the patient to say 'EE', causing adduction, or to take a deep breath, which causes abduction. The beginner will often see only the epiglottis, with a fleeting glimpse of the cords, but continued practice will allow visualization of the larynx and hypopharynx in most subjects.

In recording your findings, bear in mind that the image you see is reversed. It is advisable to label your diagram L and R in case confusion with direct examination occurs.

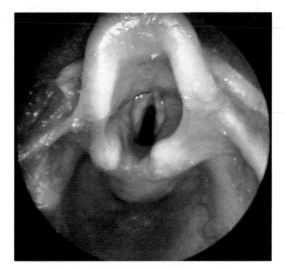

Fig. 31.3 The appearance of the larynx as seen by direct laryngoscopy.

FIBRE-OPTIC LARYNGOSCOPY

In some cases the patient will not tolerate indirect laryngoscopy, or the view of the vocal cords is obstructed by an overhanging epiglottis. In these cases, fibre-optic laryngoscopy makes examination possible without recourse to general anaesthesia. The flexible fibre-optic instrument is passed through the anaesthetized nose into the pharynx. It is then manoeuvred past the epiglottis until the interior of the larynx is seen. Although the image is smaller than that obtained by mirror examination, it allows inspection of the cords during phonation and also enables a photographic record to be made. The patient can even view his own larynx through a teaching attachment.

DIRECT LARYNGOSCOPY

Under general anaesthesia, a laryngoscope supported by some form of suspension apparatus is introduced into the larynx. With the aid of an operating microscope, a superb binocular-magnified view of the larynx is obtained and endoscopic surgery can be carried out with precision. This technique also allows the use of a carbon dioxide laser for the treatment of such lesions as papillomata and leukoplakia. Closed-circuit television, video or still photography are simple to attach to the microscope for making a record of the findings (Fig. 31.3).

CHAPTER 32

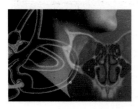

Injuries of the Larynx and Trachea

The larynx and trachea may be injured by:
1. penetrating wounds, e.g. gunshot or cut throat injuries (Fig. 32.1);
2. blunt trauma, especially from road traffic accidents;
3. inhaled flames or hot vapours;
4. swallowed corrosive poisons;
5. endotracheal tubes and inflatable cuffs.

MANAGEMENT

The diagnosis of laryngeal trauma is often missed amid other serious injuries, but should always be suspected when injury to the neck has occurred. Cricotracheal separation may not cause immediately obvious signs but may lead to asphyxia. Fractures of the larynx will produce hoarseness and stridor, and tracheostomy may be needed urgently. In cases of cut throat, it may be possible to intubate the larynx through the wound, prior to formal tracheostomy and laryngeal repair. The two priorities of treatment are:
1. to protect the airway by intubation or tracheostomy;
2. to restore laryngeal function by careful repair of the injury.

Laryngeal stenosis may result, despite repair of the larynx, and a permanent tracheostomy is sometimes necessary.

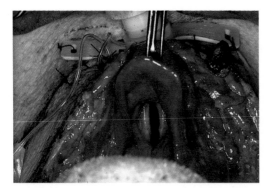

Fig. 32.1 A self-inflicted cut throat, giving a good view of the anatomy.

Various manoeuvres for the correction of laryngeal stenosis have been devised, most depending on widening the lumen with some form of skeletal graft, such as rib cartilage or the hyoid bone.

INTUBATION

A particular problem is that posed by long-term endotracheal intubation of patients on intensive care units. The avoidance of red rubber tubes and awareness of the need to control cuff pressures have led to a reduction in the incidence of stenosis, and with modern tube design, tracheostomy can usually be postponed for 2–3 weeks. Once a problem mainly limited to adult intensive-care units, there has been an increased incidence of subglottic stenosis among very premature babies as a result of improved survival rates, owing to the excellent care of neonatologists. Prolonged endotracheal ventilation for broncho-pulmonary dysplasia and respiratory distress syndrome has inevitably resulted in cases of laryngeal stenosis in tiny infants, the care of whom is highly specialized and beyond the scope of this book.

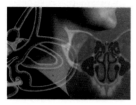

CHAPTER 33

Acute Disorders of the Larynx

Acute laryngitis—adults

Acute laryngitis is more common in winter months and is usually caused by acute coryza (common cold) or influenza. It is predisposed to by vocal over-use, smoking or drinking of spirits. If factors from both groups coexist —the heavy smoker with a cold, shouting abuse at the referee on a winter's afternoon—acute laryngitis is (fortunately for everybody else) sure to follow.

CLINICAL FEATURES

Clinical features include aphonia (the voice reduced to a whisper) or dysphonia (a painful croak) and pain around the larynx, especially on coughing.

Examination by indirect laryngoscopy shows the larynx to be red and dry, with stringy mucus between the cords.

TREATMENT

1 Total voice rest.
2 Inhalations with steam.
3 No smoking.
4 Antibiotics are rarely necessary.

Acute laryngitis—children

As a result of acute upper respiratory infection, laryngitis may develop. This may lead to airway obstruction.

CLINICAL FEATURES

1 Unwell.
2 Harsh cough.
3 Hoarse voice or aphonia.

This early stage will often respond to paracetamol and a steamy environment. If oedema develops within the limited space of the subglottis, stridor may supervene. This combination of acute laryngitis and stridor is known as croup. If there is significant or worsening airway obstruction, the child should be admitted to hospital, preferably where paediatric intensive care facilities are available.

Acute epiglottitis

More common in North America than the UK, acute epiglottitis is a localized infection of the supraglottic larynx usually by *Haemophilus influenzae*. It causes severe swelling of the epiglottis, which obstructs the laryngeal inlet. In children it constitutes the most urgent emergency—the child may progress from being perfectly well to being dead within the space of a few hours on account of airway obstruction. Fortunately, it has now become very rare in the UK because of the widespread use of HIB vaccine.

CLINICAL FEATURES

The child will become unwell, with increasing dysphagia and a quack-like cough. Stridor will develop rapidly and the child will prefer to sit up, leaning forward to ease his airway.

If the diagnosis is suspected and even though symptoms may be mild, the child should be admitted at once to hospital. At one time tracheostomy was the treatment of choice but most cases are now managed by endotracheal intubation and therapy with chloramphenicol, which will result in rapid resolution.

In adults the pain is severe and is worsened on swallowing. It is slower to develop and to resolve than in children. Respiratory obstruction is less likely to occur, but may do so with a fatal result.

Laryngotracheobronchitis

This condition occurs in infants and toddlers and is a generalized respiratory infection, probably viral in origin. In addition to laryngeal oedema, there is the production of thick tenacious secretions, which block the trachea and small airways. It is of slower onset than acute epiglottitis and there is a harsh, croupy cough. Mild cases will settle on treatment with humidified air, but more severe cases will require airway support and possible ventilation.

Laryngeal diphtheria

Laryngeal diphtheria is rarely seen now in the UK. The child is ill and usually presents the clinical picture of faucial diphtheria. Stridor suggests the spread of membrane to the larynx and trachea.

TREATMENT

1   Antitoxin.
2   General medical treatment for diphtheria.
3   Tracheostomy (q.v) may be indicated.

CHAPTER 34

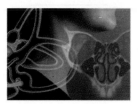

Chronic Disorders
of the Larynx

Chronic laryngitis

More common in males than females, chronic laryngitis is aggravated by:

1 habitual shouting;
2 faulty voice production coupled with excessive vocal use. Seen in teachers, actors, singers;
3 smoking;
4 spirit drinking;
5 chronic upper airway infection, such as sinusitis.

The voice is hoarse and fatigues easily. There may be discomfort and a tendency to clear the throat constantly. Examination shows the cords to be thickened and pink and the surrounding mucosa is often red and dry.

TREATMENT

Treatment is often ineffective. The voice should be rested as far as possible, any upper airway sepsis dealt with and steam inhalations given to humidify the larynx. Voice therapy may be helpful in cases of faulty voice production and referral to a singing teacher is of value to professional or amateur singers.

Hyperkeratosis of the larynx

Hyperkeratosis of the larynx may supervene upon chronic laryngitis. The cords become covered in white plaques of keratinized epithelium, which may become florid. Histology shows dysplasia, which may progress to malignancy, and the plaques should be removed for histology.

Vocal cord nodules

Vocal cord nodules (singer's nodes) occur most commonly in children and result from excessive vocal use. The appearance is of a small, smooth nodule on the free edge of each cord, composed of fibrous tissue covered with epithelium. Removal by microlaryngoscopy followed by voice rest may be necessary but most cases respond to speech therapy.

Tuberculosis of the larynx

Tuberculosis of the larynx is now very rare and occurs only in the presence of pulmonary tuberculosis. Hoarseness occurs as a result of tuberculous granulations and agonizing dysphagia may follow. Treatment is by antituberculous drugs.

Syphilitic laryngitis

Syphilitic laryngitis is also extremely rare but the possibility of a gumma must be considered in cases of chronic hoarseness. Malignant change may also be present.

NB. Any case of persistent hoarseness must be considered malignant until examination and, if necessary, biopsy have excluded such a cause.

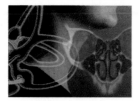

CHAPTER 35

Tumours of the Larynx

BENIGN TUMOURS

Benign tumours of the larynx are rare and cause persistent hoarseness. The commonest tumours encountered are:

1 papilloma — solitary or multiple;
2 haemangioma — almost exclusively in infants;
3 fibroma.

Papillomata and haemangiomata are considered in more detail in Chapter 37.

MALIGNANT TUMOURS

PATHOLOGY

Malignant tumours of the larynx are virtually always squamous cell carcinoma. Adenoid cystic carcinoma and sarcoma may occur on rare occasions.

AETIOLOGY

Malignant tumours are commoner in males by a ratio of 10:1, occurring almost exclusively in smokers. The peak age incidence is 55–65 years, but it can occur in young adults.

Glottic carcinoma (60% of cases)

The prime symptom of glottic carcinoma (Fig. 35.1) is hoarseness, which may persist as the only symptom for many months. Only when spread from the cord has occurred will earache, dysphagia and dyspnoea supervene.

Supraglottic carcinoma (30% of cases)

Supraglottic carcinoma, as well as producing a change in the voice, may metastasize early to the cervical nodes.

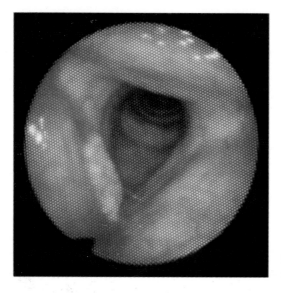

Fig. 35.1 Early glottic carcinoma.

Subglottic carcinoma

Subglottic carcinoma produces less hoarseness but increasing airway obstruction. It must not be mistaken for asthma or chronic bronchitis.

SPREAD OF LARYNGEAL CARCINOMA

Spread is local initially and proceeds:

1   along the cord to the anterior commissure and onto the opposite cord;
2   upwards onto the ventricular band and epiglottis;
3   downwards to the subglottis;
4   deeply into the laryngeal muscles, causing cord fixation.

Lymphatic spread from glottic lesions is late, but occurs readily from supraglottic and subglottic sites to the deep cervical nodes.

Pulmonary metastases occur occasionally but other distant metastases are rare.

DIAGNOSIS

Every case of hoarseness should be examined by indirect laryngoscopy; malignant growths are usually seen easily. Diagnosis is confirmed by microlaryngoscopy and biopsy.

The chest must be X-rayed as bronchial carcinoma also may be present. CT scanning of the larynx is often helpful in defining the extent of spread, and is usually performed prior to deciding on treatment.

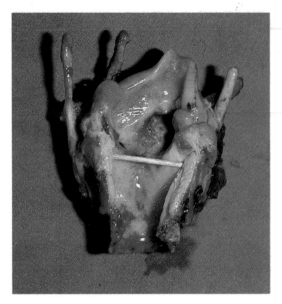

Fig. 35.2 Laryngectomy specimen opened from posteriorly, showing a left-sided carcinoma.

TREATMENT

1 Radiotherapy by external radiation is usually employed. In a small tumour limited to one cord (the stage at which it should be diagnosed), the 5-year survival rate is 80–90% and the patient retains a normal larynx.

2 In very extensive disease or if there is recurrence following radiotherapy, total laryngectomy is necessary (Fig. 35.2). The patient obviously then has a permanent tracheostomy and will need to develop oesophageal speech. Good oesophageal speech is attained by about 30% of patients; a further 30% develop reasonable voice but the remainder never manage more than a mouthed whisper.

Many patients are now provided with a tracheopharyngeal valve. A fistula is formed between the trachea and pharynx and a prosthetic valve fitted to the fistula. Occlusion by the finger of the tracheostomy allows air to flow into the hypopharynx, while vibration of the soft tissue produces phonation. This then allows fluent lung-powered voice for the laryngectomee.

Rehabilitation following laryngectomy concentrates on the development of speech with help from the speech therapist, but also requires training in looking after the tracheostomy, changing the tube as necessary and developing confidence socially after mutilating surgery.

PROGNOSIS

Glottic carcinoma diagnosed early and treated effectively is virtually a curable disease. The later the diagnosis is made, the worse the prognosis. *Never neglect hoarseness.*

Supraglottic and subglottic tumours have a poorer prognosis owing to the likelihood of rather later development of symptoms and early nodal spread. About 10% of all patients successfully treated for laryngeal cancer will subsequently develop carcinoma of the bronchus.

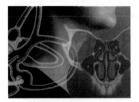

CHAPTER 36

Vocal Cord Paralysis

Nerve supply of the laryngeal muscles

All the intrinsic muscles of the larynx, with the exception of the crico-thyroids, are supplied by the recurrent laryngeal nerves.

The cricothyroids, which act as tensors of the cords, are supplied by external branches of the superior laryngeal nerves.

Semon's law

In a progressive lesion of the recurrent laryngeal nerves, the abductors are paralysed before the adductors. Thus, in incomplete paralysis, the cord will be brought to the midline by the adductors, but in complete paralysis it falls away to the paramedian position. Semon's law is not fully understood, but may reflect the fact that the adductor muscles are much more powerful than the abductors.

Recurrent laryngeal nerve palsy (Figs 36.1 and 36.2)

The left recurrent laryngeal nerve has a long course, extending down into the chest before recurring around the arch of the aorta to return to the larynx. It is therefore more susceptible to disease than the shorter right recurrent nerve, which turns around the subclavian artery.

The voice in recurrent nerve palsy is weak and breathy, and the cough is ineffective. As compensation by the opposite cord occurs, the voice improves.

The causes of *left* recurrent nerve palsy in the chest are:

1 carcinoma of the bronchus;
2 carcinoma of the oesophagus;
3 malignant mediastinal nodes;
4 aortic aneurysm;
5 cardiac and oesophageal surgery.

The causes of paralysis of the *right* or *left* recurrent nerve in the neck are:

1 thyroid surgery;
2 carcinoma of the thyroid gland;
3 carcinoma of the hypopharynx and oesophagus;

CORDS IN FULL ABDUCTION

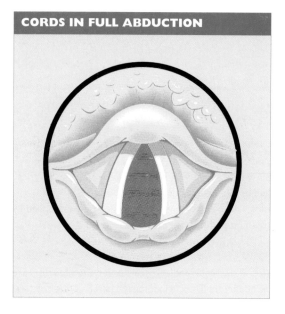

Fig. 36.1 The cords in full abduction during inspiration.

LEFT RECURRENT NERVE PALSY ON PHONATION

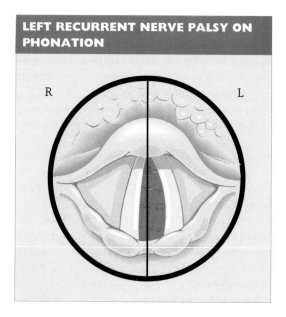

Fig. 36.2 Left recurrent nerve palsy on phonation (mirror view). Note the persisting glottic aperture owing to the inability of the left cord to move to the midline.

4 cervical spine surgery (Cloward's operation);

5 penetrating wounds;

6 mediastinoscopy.

Some cases of recurrent nerve palsy are idiopathic or may follow viral infections, such as influenza.

Bilateral recurrent laryngeal nerve palsy

Bilateral recurrent laryngeal nerve palsy occurs most commonly following surgery or malignancy of the thyroid gland, but may be the result of pseudobulbar palsy. Because the cords lie near the midline, the airway is impaired and tracheostomy may be necessary.

Combined vagal and recurrent nerve palsy

Combined vagal and recurrent nerve palsy occurs in lesions of the medulla or vagus trunk.

1 Medulla—neoplasm, vascular lesions, syringobulbia, bulbar poliomyelitis.

2 Vagus trunk—tumours of the skull base, e.g. carcinoma of the nasopharynx; tumours of the jugular foramen—glomus jugulare tumour; chemodectoma of the vagus.

Functional aphonia

Functional aphonia is a condition found mostly in teenaged females and is psychogenic. The voice is reduced to a whisper, examination shows weak adduction of the cords but sound is produced normally on coughing. Treatment lies in the realm of the communication therapist or psychotherapy.

Treatment of vocal cord paralysis

The first step is always to try to identify the cause.

Bilateral cord palsy will probably produce stridor and urgent tracheostomy may be required. The airway can be improved by arytenoidectomy, but the voice will be worse as a result.

The voice can be improved in cases of unilateral cord palsy by the endoscopic injection of a suspension of microspheres of inert plastic material alongside the paralysed cord. This will move the paralysed cord medially and allow the opposite cord to meet its fellow. Improvement in voice quality results. It will also restore laryngeal competence and improve the ability to cough effectively. It is a very good palliation in cases of carcinoma of the bronchus. For unilateral vocal cord palsy of a cause compatible with survival, the operation of vocal cord medialization is available. A window is cut in the thyroid cartilage and a block of silastic inserted to displace the cord towards the mid line. It has the advantage of being reversible if the cord palsy should recover. Functional aphonia is usually self-limiting, or responds to explanation and encouragement. The help of the speech therapist is valuable in persistent cases and some patients may require psychiatric treatment.

CHAPTER 37

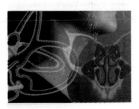

Airway Obstruction in Infants and Children

Upper airway obstruction in children is dangerous and may progress rapidly. It is essential to make a firm diagnosis and take the appropriate action without delay.

SIGNS OF AIRWAY OBSTRUCTION

1 Stertor is the noise produced by obstruction in the throat, i.e. above the larynx, and is usually a low-pitched choking type of noise.

2 Stridor is a high-pitched sound produced by narrowing within the more rigid confines of the larynx or trachea. In laryngeal obstruction the stridor is inspiratory; in tracheal lesions it is usually both inspiratory and expiratory.

3 Use of accessory muscles of respiration.

4 Pallor, sweating and restlessness.

5 Tachycardia.

6 Cyanosis. It is important to examine the child in adequate lighting, preferably daylight. The lips particularly will show the dusky coloration, which may be very subtle.

7 Intercostal and sternal recession (Fig. 37.1). The sternum may be sucked in almost to the vertebrae in the child's attempts to breathe.

8 Exhaustion—a late stage in asphyxia, which should be avoided. The child makes less effort to breathe, stridor and insuction become less pronounced and apnoea is not far off.

Box 37.1 Signs of airway obstruction.

Management of airway obstruction

The management of airway insufficiency always depends on the severity of the obstruction, and severe obstruction necessitates immediate airway support by oxygen, endotracheal intubation or even tracheostomy.

If time and the child's condition allow, every child with stridor should have a PA chest X-ray and a lateral soft-tissue film of the neck, which will show the larynx and upper trachea clearly. If a vascular ring or tracheo-oesophageal fistula is suspected, a barium swallow is a necessary investigation.

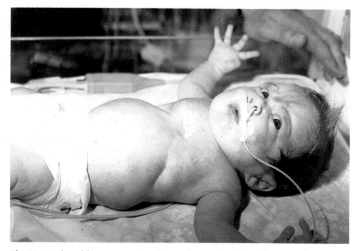

Fig. 37.1 Baby with severe upper airway obstruction. Note the sternal recession and paradoxical abdominal movement.

Neonates may be intubated without the need for general anaesthesia but great care must be taken not to damage the larynx and cause further obstruction from haematoma or oedema. Older children, unless so anoxic as to be unconscious, will require general anaesthesia for intubation, and at the same time the larynx, trachea and bronchi should be inspected. The diagnosis is then usually apparent and further management can be directed appropriately.

LARYNGOSCOPY AND BRONCHOSCOPY

Inspection of the airways in cases of respiratory obstruction calls for the highest degree of cooperation between surgeon and anaesthetist.

The larynx is inspected under deep anaesthesia using a rigid paediatric laryngoscope and Hopkins rod telescope (Fig. 37.2). An anaesthetic type laryngoscope usually gives an inadequate view owing to its poorer lighting.

Bronchoscopy in babies and children has been facilitated greatly by the introduction of ventilating bronchoscopes, which allow coupling to a T-piece anaesthetic circuit and at the same time provide superb vision through a rod-lens telescope system (Fig. 37.3). A side channel allows for instrumentation and suction. Using this type of bronchoscope, the airways of even small premature babies may be examined with a much greater degree of precision and safety than is possible with the older type open bronchoscope tube.

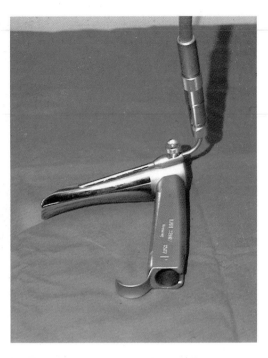

Fig. 37.2 A small laryngoscope used for examining young children.

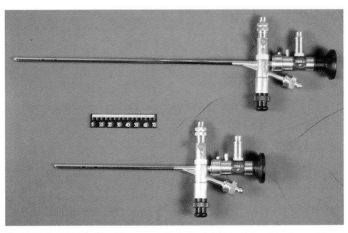

Fig. 37.3 Ventilating bronchoscopes. Note the telescope, the side channel for instrumentation and the inlet for anaesthetic gases and oxygen.

Causes of upper airway obstruction in infancy

SUPRA LARYNGEAL CAUSES

Choanal atresia

Failure of posterior canalization of the nasal airways results in severe neonatal airway obstruction, which is relieved by crying. Surgical correction will be required.

Micrognathia

Underdevelopment of the mandible as in Pierre Robin syndrome or Treacher–Collins syndrome results in posterior displacement of the tongue and oropharyngeal obstruction. The neonate may asphyxiate unless corrective measures are taken.

Adeno-tonsillar hypertrophy

Large tonsils and adenoids may occlude the naso-oro-pharyngeal airway to a serious degree, especially during sleep. This may result in obstructive apnoea during sleep, with loud snoring punctuated by periods of silence followed by a large gasp. If not recognized and treated, right heart failure may ensue.

LARYNGEAL CAUSES

Congenital

Laryngomalacia (Fig. 37.4)

The stridor starts at or shortly after birth and is due to inward collapse of the soft laryngeal tissues on inspiration. It usually resolves by the age of 2 or 3 years, but meanwhile the baby may have real respiratory difficulties. Diagnosis is confirmed by laryngoscopy without intubation when the supraglottic collapse is seen on inspiration. It can be relieved by division or excision of the aryepiglottic folds.

Congenital subglottic stenosis

This occurs at the level of the cricoid cartilage. There will be stridor from birth and the stenosis may be visible on a lateral X-ray of the neck. Diagnosis is confirmed by laryngoscopy.

Laryngeal webs

Laryngeal webs are anteriorly situated (Fig. 37.5) and if large can cause

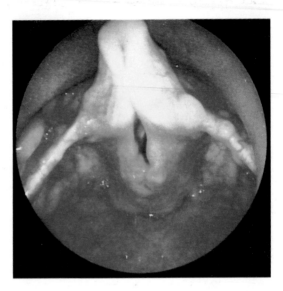

Fig. 37.4 Laryngomalacia. Note the insuction of the supraglottic structures, causing airway narrowing.

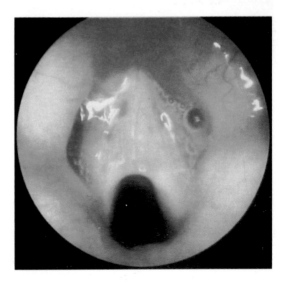

Fig. 37.5 Anterior laryngeal web.

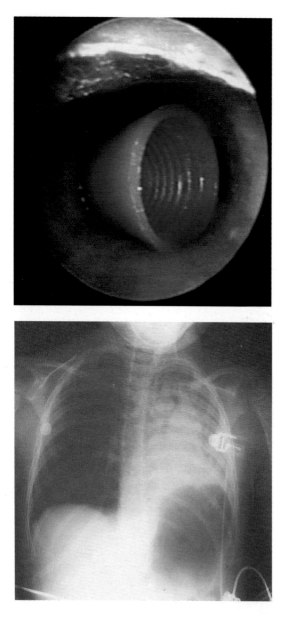

Fig. 37.6 Part of a ball-point pen lodged in the left main bronchus as seen at bronchoscopy. The chest film shows loss of lung volume and mediastinal shift.

severe stridor and obstruction. The most extreme degree of webbing, atresia, is fatal unless immediate tracheostomy is performed.

Laryngeal cysts
Laryngeal cysts may be congenital or may be the result of endotracheal intubation. They may cause variable airway obstruction, often dependent on position.

Vascular ring
A vascular ring developmental anomaly of the aorta — surrounds the oesophagus and trachea, causing constriction. Diagnosis is made by barium swallow and angiography, and the treatment is by surgery to divide the vascular ring.

Acquired

Foreign body (Figs 37.6 and 37.7)
The sudden onset of stridor in a formerly normal child must always be regarded as being due to a foreign body until proved otherwise. A history of choking and coughing, especially if while eating, should alert the attending doctor to the likelihood of aspiration; peanuts are particularly dangerous in this respect and should *never* be given to youngsters. Examination and chest X-rays may be entirely normal and the only way to exclude a foreign body in the bronchus is by bronchoscopy.

A larger foreign body may lodge in the larynx and cause severe respiratory distress. It may be possible to remove it by the Heimlich manoeuvre (compression of the upper abdomen to raise intrathoracic pressure) but if this fails, endoscopy or tracheostomy will be necessary.

Acute laryngitis, acute epiglottitis and laryngotracheobronchitis
Described in Chapter 33.

Subglottic stenosis (Fig. 37.8)
Subglottic stenosis is now seen most commonly in low-birth-weight babies who have required prolonged ventilation by endotracheal tube, but may occur at any age from intubation or trauma. Treatment is highly specialized and entails some form of laryngotracheoplasty. Subglottic stenosis cannot always be avoided.

Multiple laryngeal papillomata (Fig. 37.9)
Multiple laryngeal papillomata should be suspected in a child with progressive hoarseness or aphonia and airway obstruction. There may be little

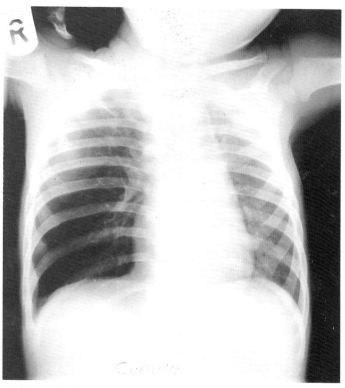

Fig. 37.7 Foreign body in the right main bronchus in a baby of 6 months. Note that the right lung is hyperinflated and therefore darker on the X-ray.

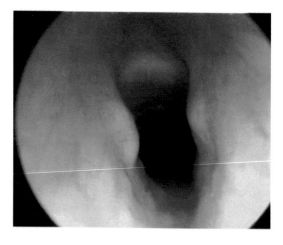

Fig. 37.8 Endoscopic view showing moderate subglottic stenosis and small ductal cysts following ventilation as a neonate.

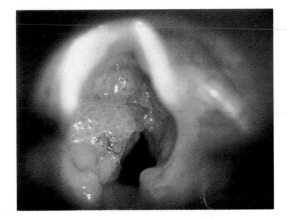

Fig. 37.9 A large mass of papillomata on the left vocal cord.

stridor since the mass of papillomata is too soft to vibrate the air column. Diagnosis is by direct laryngoscopy, and removal of the papillomata is best accomplished using the carbon dioxide laser, which is very accurate and, if used carefully, causes least damage. The papillomata are of viral origin (HPV 6 or 11) and have a strong tendency to recur.

NB. Any child with stridor is potentially at risk of dying from asphyxia and every case should be investigated to determine the cause. It is dangerous to believe that all children 'grow out' of a tendency to stridor.

CHAPTER 38

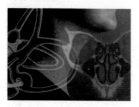

Conditions of the Hypopharynx

FOREIGN BODIES

Fish, poultry and other bones are often swallowed inadvertently. Usually they will scratch or tear the pharyngeal mucosa before passing down into the stomach. However, they may on occasions lodge in the hypopharynx or oesophagus, where they may lead to perforation, mediastinitis or abscess, or even fatal perforation of the aorta. Children and the mentally disturbed may swallow coins, toys or more bizarre objects (Fig. 38.1) and the elderly may swallow their dentures.

MANAGEMENT

It may be very difficult for the casualty officer or novice ENT surgeon to decide whether a foreign body has simply caused an abrasion and has passed on, or is impacted. The following routine should be adopted.

1   Take a careful history, noting the nature of the suspected foreign body (is it radio-opaque?) and the time of ingestion.

2   Examine the pharynx and larynx, paying particular attention to the tonsils and valleculae. (Fish bones often stick here.) A foreign body lodged in the cervical oesophagus will cause pain on pressing the larynx against the spine.

3   X-ray the chest and neck (lateral view) — remember that fish bones and plastic are likely to be radiolucent and may not show.

4   If marked dysphagia is present, or a foreign body is seen on X-ray, oesophagoscopy is indicated.

5   If symptoms persist despite normal X-ray appearances, oesophagoscopy is necessary to exclude a foreign body.

The potential gravity of an impacted foreign body cannot be overemphasized, and if there is any doubt, expert advice must be sought.

Post-cricoid web

The Paterson–Brown Kelly syndrome (later described by Plummer and Vinson) usually occurs in middle-aged women but can occur in males, though rarely. It is associated with iron-deficiency anaemia and the develop-

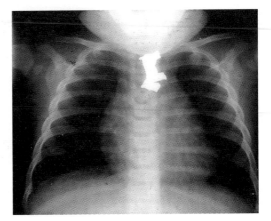

Fig. 38.1 Man eats dog.

ment of a postcricoid web. The features of iron deficiency (glossitis, angular stomatitis and microcytic anaemia) will be present and the web will be demonstrated by barium swallow.

TREATMENT

The iron deficiency is corrected by iron supplements and the web is dilated periodically. A small number of patients with this condition will go on to develop postcricoid carcinoma.

PHARYNGEAL POUCH (PHARYNGEAL DIVERTICULUM)

The pharyngeal mucosa herniates between the oblique and transverse fibres of the inferior constrictor muscle to produce a persistent pouch (Fig. 38.2). The condition occurs almost exclusively in the elderly and is thought to be due to failure of the cricopharyngeus part of the inferior constrictor to relax during swallowing, thus building up pressure above it.

CLINICAL FEATURES

1 Discomfort in the throat initially.
2 Dysphagia as the pouch enlarges.
3 Regurgitation of undigested food.
4 Aspiration pneumonia if untreated.
5 Gurgling noises in the throat on swallowing or pressure on the neck.
NB. A pouch almost never causes a palpable neck swelling.

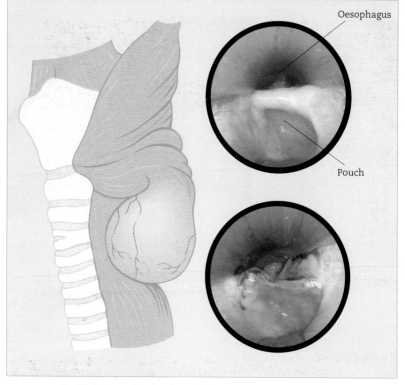

Oesophagus

Pouch

Fig. 38.2 External and endoscopic views of the pharyngeal pouch. The photographs show appearances before and after endoscopic diverticulotomy with a stapling device.

INVESTIGATION

The pouch is revealed by barium swallow (Fig. 38.3).

TREATMENT

1 The early case can be managed by periodic dilatation of the cricopharyngeus.

2 An established pouch causing symptoms will require surgical treatment. Under general anaesthesia, a dilating rigid pharyngoscope is used to demonstrate the party wall between the oesophagus anteriorly and the pouch posteriorly. A staple gun is then used to divide the wall and at the same time staple the cut edges (Fig. 38.2). The patient is usually able to eat the following day and the hospital stay is very short.

3 Only rarely is it now necessary to excise a pouch by external approach through the neck.

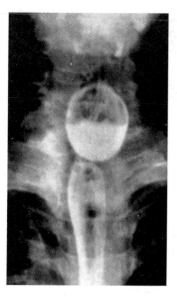
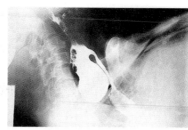

(b)

Fig. 38.3 A barium swallow X-ray showing a pharyngeal pouch (left); lateral view (right).

MALIGNANT DISEASE OF THE HYPOPHARYNX

Malignant disease of the hypopharynx occurs in two main forms.

1 Carcinoma of the piriform fossa—predominantly a disease of males (Fig. 38.4).

2 Post-cricoid carcinoma—predominantly a disease of females (Fig. 38.5). This may supervene on long-standing Paterson–Brown Kelly syndrome.

CLINICAL FEATURES

1 Increasing dysphagia and weight loss.

2 An enlarged cervical node due to metastasis may be the first complaint of a patient with a small hypopharyngeal cancer not yet large enough to produce dysphagia.

3 Hoarseness may be present from involvement of the recurrent laryngeal nerve or direct spread to the larynx.

4 Referred otalgia is often present, especially on swallowing.

5 Mirror examination may reveal the malignant ulcer, or pooling of saliva in the hypopharynx.

Spread occurs locally by direct invasion, but nodal metastases in the neck occur early in the course of the disease. Distant metastases sometimes occur (compare with laryngeal carcinoma).

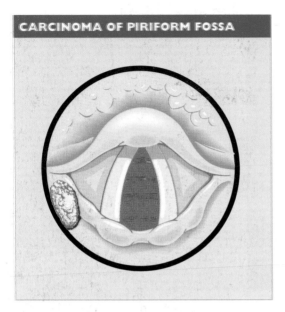

Fig. 38.4 Carcinoma of the piriform fossa.

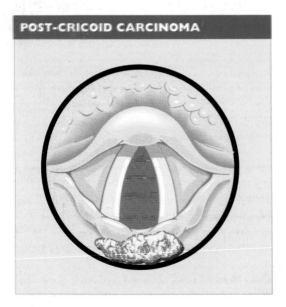

Fig. 38.5 Post-cricoid carcinoma.

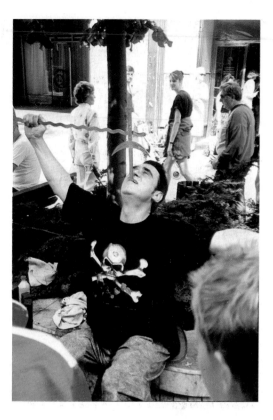

Fig. 38.6 A sword swallower in Prague. The first ever oesophagoscopy was performed in the 19th century on a sword swallower by Küssmaul to demonstrate its feasibility.

INVESTIGATIONS

Every case of dysphagia must be investigated by barium swallow and oesophagoscopy. Even if the X-ray is normal, direct examination must be performed in the presence of dysphagia.

TREATMENT

1   Hypopharyngeal cancers are usually treated by pharyngolaryngectomy, a major operation with a definite mortality. Repair of the pharynx is difficult and accomplished either by stomach pull-up or by the use of vascularized skin flaps. The use of a free graft of jejunum with microvascular anastomosis has been shown to be effective and is a less severe operation than stomach pull-up, though with less certain results. The 5-year survival rate is of the order of 35%.

2   Radiotherapy may produce cure or good palliation but the patient will suffer considerable discomfort during the course of treatment and should be warned accordingly.

3   Many cases are unfortunately untreatable when first diagnosed and no effort must be spared to relieve the patient's misery with analgesics, tranquillizers and devoted nursing care.

GLOBUS PHARYNGIS

Globus pharyngis is the term applied to the sensation of a lump or discomfort in the throat, probably owing to cricopharyngeal spasm. The discomfort is relieved by eating and there is no interference with the swallowing of food or liquids.

The symptoms tend to be aggravated by the patient's constant action of swallowing, and frequently introspection and anxiety add to the problem. A proportion of patients with globus pharyngis will be found to have reflux oesphagitis or a gastric ulcer and a barium swallow should always be performed, both to find such conditions and to exclude as far as possible organic pathology in the throat. Many cases have a psychological cause and are aggravated by anxiety and introspection.

If symptoms persist, oesophagoscopy is essential—a normal barium swallow does not rule out organic disease.

If no organic cause for the symptoms exists, most patients improve with reassurance reinforced by adequate examination and investigation. A short course of tranquillizers is often helpful.

CHAPTER 39

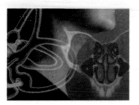

Tracheostomy

Tracheostomy, the making of an opening into the trachea, has been practised since the first century BC, and is a procedure with which all doctors should be familiar.

INDICATIONS

Indications for tracheostomy may be classified as follows:
1 conditions causing upper airway obstruction;
2 conditions necessitating protection of the tracheobronchial tree;
3 conditions causing respiratory failure.

Protection of the tracheobronchial tube

Any condition causing pharyngeal or laryngeal incompetence may allow aspiration of food, saliva, blood or gastric contents. If the condition is of short duration, e.g. general anaesthesia, endotracheal intubation is appropriate, but for chronic conditions tracheostomy is necessary. It allows easy access to the trachea and bronchi for regular suction and permits the use of a cuffed tube, which affords further protection against aspiration. Examples of such conditions are:
1 polyneuritis (e.g. Guillain–Barré syndrome);
2 bulbar poliomyelitis;
3 multiple sclerosis;
4 myasthenia gravis;
5 tetanus;
6 brain-stem stroke;
7 coma due to:
　(a) head injury;
　(b) poisoning;
　(c) stroke;
　(d) cerebral tumour;
　(e) intracranial surgery (unless the state of coma is likely to be prolonged, endotracheal intubation is preferable in the first place);
8 multiple facial fractures.

UPPER AIRWAY OBSTRUCTION

Congenital
1   Subglottic or upper tracheal stenosis.
2   Laryngeal web.
3   Laryngeal and vallecular cysts.
4   Tracheo-oesophageal anomalies.
5   Haemangioma of larynx.

Trauma
1   Prolonged endotracheal intubation.
2   Gunshot wounds and cut throat, laryngeal fracture.
3   Inhalation of steam or hot vapour.
4   Swallowing of corrosive fluids.
5   Radiotherapy (may cause oedema).

Infections
1   Acute epiglottitis (see Chapter 33).
2   Laryngotracheobronchitis.
3   Diphtheria.
4   Ludwig's angina.

Malignant tumours
1   Advanced malignant disease of the tongue, larynx, pharynx or upper trachea.
2   As part of a surgical procedure for the treatment of laryngeal cancer.
3   Carcinoma of thyroid.

Bilateral laryngeal paralysis
1   Following thyroidectomy.
2   Bulbar palsy.
3   Following oesophageal or heart surgery.

Foreign body
1   Remember the Heimlich manoeuvre — grasp the patient from behind with a fist in the epigastrium and apply sudden pressure upwards towards the diaphragm. It may need to be repeated several times before the foreign body is expelled.

Box 39.1 Upper airway obstruction.

Respiratory failure

Tracheostomy in cases of respiratory failure allows:
1   reduction of dead space by about 70 mL (in the adult);
2   bypass of laryngeal resistance;
3   access to the trachea for the removal of bronchial secretions;
4   administration of humidified oxygen;
5   positive-pressure ventilation when necessary.
Respiratory failure is often multifactorial and may be considered under the following headings.

1   Pulmonary disease—exacerbation of chronic bronchitis and emphysema; severe asthma; postoperative pneumonia from accumulated secretions.

2   Abnormalities of the thoracic cage—severe chest injury (flail chest); ankylosing spondylitis; severe kyphosis.

3   Neuromuscular dysfunction—e.g. Guillain–Barré syndrome; tetanus; motor neurone disease; poliomyelitis.

Criteria for performing tracheostomy

Tracheostomy should, whenever possible, be carried out as an elective procedure and not as a desperate last resort. There are degrees of urgency.

1   If the patient has life-threatening airway obstruction when first seen, it is obvious that urgent treatment is required. If endotracheal intubation fails, tracheostomy must be done at once. There is no time for sterility—with the left hand, hold the trachea on either side to immobilize it, make a vertical incision through the tissues of the neck into the trachea and twist the blade through 90° to open up the trachea. There will be copious dark bleeding but the patient will gasp air through the opening. Using the index finger of the left hand as a guide in the wound, try to insert some sort of tube into the trachea. The blood should then be sucked out by whatever means are available. Once an airway is established, the tracheostomy can be tidied up under more controlled conditions.

2   In patients with airway obstruction of more gradual onset, do not allow the situation to deteriorate to that described above. Stridor, recession and tachycardia denote the need for intervention, and cyanosis and bradycardia indicate that you are running out of time. The case should be discussed with an experienced anaesthetist, and the patient taken to the operating theatre. The ideal is to carry out tracheostomy under general anaesthesia with endotracheal intubation. Once a tube has been inserted, the airway is safe and the tracheostomy can be performed calmly and carefully with full sterile precautions. If the anaesthetist is unable to intubate the patient, it will be necessary to perform the operation under local anaesthetic using infiltration with lignocaine. The anaesthetist meanwhile will administer oxygen through a face-mask.

3   Elective tracheostomy should be carried out before deterioration occurs in non-obstructive cases as listed above and patients who have previously been intubated because of obstruction or for ventilation but who cannot be extubated safely.

Such elective tracheostomy cases are ideal for trainees to learn the technique of the operation safely under supervision and every such opportunity should be taken.

Dictum

In cases of respiratory obstruction and respiratory failure and in the absence of steady improvement, support the airway by tracheostomy or endotracheal intubation.

Remember that children may deteriorate with dramatic suddenness.

THE OPERATION OF ELECTIVE TRACHEOSTOMY

Like any other operation, tracheostomy can be learned only by instruction and practice, so that only a brief description will be given.

The operation should be carried out under general anaesthesia with endotracheal intubation. The neck should be extended and the head must be straight, not turned to one side. A transverse incision is preferable to a vertical incision, and should be centred midway between the cricoid carti-lage and sternal notch (Fig. 39.1). The strap muscles are identified and re-tracted laterally (Fig. 39.2) and the thyroid isthmus is divided. Once the trachea has been reached (it is always deeper than you expect), the cricoid must be identified by palpation and the tracheal rings counted. An opening is made into the trachea, centred on the third and fourth rings (Fig. 39.3). In adults, an ellipse of sufficient size to accept the tracheostomy tube is excised, but in children, a single slit in the tracheal wall is preferable, after

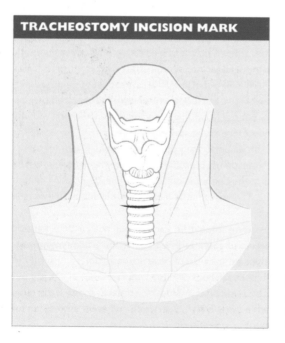

TRACHEOSTOMY INCISION MARK

Fig. 39.1 Tracheostomy showing the land marks of the neck and the incision for operation.

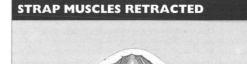

STRAP MUSCLES RETRACTED

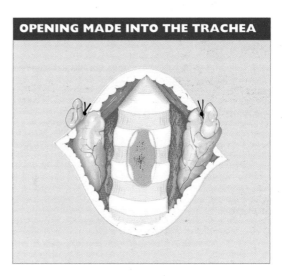

Fig. 39.2 The strap muscles are retracted, exposing the trachea and the thyroid isthmus.

OPENING MADE INTO THE TRACHEA

Fig. 39.3 The thyroid isthmus has been divided and an opening made in the anterior tracheal wall.

first inserting stay sutures on either side to allow traction on the opening in order to insert the tube.

After insertion of the tracheostomy tube, the trachea is aspirated thoroughly and unless the skin incision has been excessively long it is left unsutured. To sew the wound tightly makes surgical emphysema more likely and replacement of the tube more difficult.

Choice of tracheostomy tube

The choice of tube depends on the reason for the tracheostomy.

1 In cases of airway obstruction, a silver tube such as the Negus is ideal. It has an inner tube, which can be removed for cleaning, and has an expiratory flap-valve (sometimes called a speaking valve) to allow phonation.

2 In cases requiring ventilation or protection from aspirated secretions, a cuffed tube is necessary. The day of the red rubber tube has gone, and inert plastic tubes are now used. The cuff should be of a low-pressure design to prevent stricture formation.

3 Small children should never be fitted with a cuffed tube because of the risk of causing stenosis. A plain silastic tube should be used initially, and if ventilation is not required it can be changed at a later date to a silver tube fitted with an optionally valved inner tube (e.g. Sheffield tracheostomy tube). It is beyond the scope of this book to consider in detail the indications for metal or plastic tubes.

After-care of the tracheostomy

Nursing care

Nursing care must be of the highest standard to keep the tube patent and prevent dislodgement.

Position

Adult patients in the postoperative period should usually be sitting well propped up; care must be taken in infants that the chin does not occlude the tracheostomy and the neck should be extended slightly over a rolled-up towel.

Suction

Suction is applied at regular intervals dictated by the amount of secretions present. A clean catheter must be passed down into the tube in conscious patients. Unconscious or ventilated patients will require deeper suction and physiotherapy.

Humidification

Humidification of the inspired air is essential to prevent drying and the formation of crusts and is achieved by any conventional humidifier. Remember that the humidity you can see is due to water droplets, not vapour, and may waterlog small infants.

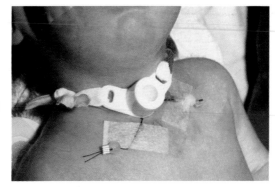

Fig. 39.4 A newly performed tracheostomy in a small child. Note the stay sutures on either side to aid replacement of the tube should it become dislodged.

Avoidance of crusts

Avoidance of crusts is aided by adequate humidification; if necessary, sterile saline (1 mL) can be introduced into the trachea, followed by suction.

Tube changing

Tube changing should be avoided if possible for 2 or 3 days, after which the track should be well established and the tube can be changed easily. Meanwhile, if a silver tube has been inserted, the inner tube can be removed and cleaned as often as necessary. Cuffed tubes need particular attention, with regular deflation of the cuff to prevent pressure necrosis. The amount of air in the cuff should be the minimum required to prevent an air leak.

Decannulation

Decannulation should only be carried out when it is obvious that the tracheostomy is no longer required. The patient should be able to manage with the tube occluded for at least 24 h before it is removed (Fig. 39.4). Decannulation in children often presents particular difficulties. After decannulation, the patient should remain in hospital under observation for several days.

Complications

Periochondritis and subglottic stenosis

Periochondritis and subglottic stenosis may result, especially if the cricoid cartilage is injured. Go below the first ring.

Mediastinal emphysema or pneumothorax

Mediastinal emphysema or pneumothorax may occur after a very low tracheostomy, or if the tube becomes displaced into the pretracheal space. The chest should be X-rayed after operation.

Obstruction

Obstruction of the tube or trachea by crusts of inspissated secretion may prove to be fatal. If the airway becomes obstructed and cannot be cleared by suction, act boldly. Remove the whole tube and replace it if blocked. If the tube is patent, explore the trachea with angled forceps to remove the obstruction. An explosive cough may expel the crust and the tube can then be replaced.

Complete dislodgement

Complete dislodgement of the tube may occur if it is not adequately fixed. Hold the wound edges apart with a tracheal dilator and put in a clean tube. A good light is essential.

Partial dislodgement

Partial dislodgement of the tube is more difficult to recognize and may be fatal. The tube comes to lie in front of the trachea, the airway will be impaired and, if left, erosion of the innominate artery may result in catastrophic haemorrhage. Make sure that at all times the patient breathes freely through the tube, and such an occurrence should be avoided. Surgical emphysema of startling severity may occur if the patient is on positive-pressure ventilation.

It is common experience that as soon as a tracheostomy has been performed there is pressure from all concerned to close it. A tracheostomy must be retained until you are sure it is no longer necessary.

CHAPTER 40

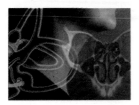

Diseases of the Salivary Glands

The salivary glands consist of:

1   the parotid glands;
2   the submandibular glands;
3   minor salivary glands throughout the mouth and upper air passages. (The sublingual collection is included in this group.)

Parotid gland

The parotid gland lies on the side of the face in close relationship to the ear, the angle of the mandible and styloid muscles. The facial nerve enters the posterior pole of the parotid gland and divides within its substance into its various branches, which exit at the anterior margin of the gland. It is the presence of the facial nerve within the parotid that makes surgery of this gland so difficult. Its duct opens opposite the second upper molar tooth, where it forms a small visible papilla. Its secretomotor nerve supply comes from the glossopharyngeal nerve via the tympanic plexus in the middle ear.

The saliva produced is entirely serous. The surface outline of the gland is shown in Fig. 40.1.

The submandibular salivary gland

The submandibular gland lies in the floor of the mouth below and medial to the mandible and its greater part is external to the mylohyoid muscle. The deep part of the gland curves around the back of the mylohyoid and the duct runs forwards to open at the sublingual papilla. The deep part of the gland lies on the lingual nerve, from which it receives its secretomotor supply derived from the facial nerve via the chorda tympani in the middle ear. The saliva from the submandibular gland is both serous and mucous.

The minor salivary glands

The minor salivary glands can be seen and felt in the lips, cheeks, palate and upper air passages. They produce mainly mucous saliva (remember the noun is *mucus*) and are responsible for a large proportion of the total saliva secreted. They are subject to many of the diseases that affect the major salivary glands.

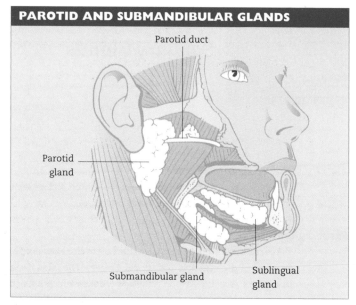

PAROTID AND SUBMANDIBULAR GLANDS

Parotid duct

Parotid gland

Submandibular gland

Sublingual gland

Fig. 40.1 The surface outline of the parotid and submandibular glands. The parotid gland is larger than is usually appreciated.

HISTORY-TAKING—SALIENT POINTS

In asking the history, enquire particularly about pain and swelling of the glands in relation to eating. If the duct is obstructed, the whole gland will become tense and painful and enlarge visibly during saliva production, and will resolve slowly over about an hour.

If a lump is present, ask about variation in size and whether it is related to food. Tumours do not enlarge during salivation, but do tend to get bigger with the passage of time.

Ask about dryness of the mouth, remembering that obstruction of even two major glands produces little apparent change. Persistent dryness suggests diffuse salivary gland disease.

Ask about recent contact with mumps.

EXAMINATION OF THE SALIVARY GLANDS

First, inspect the salivary glands externally, noting any swellings or asymmetry. The function of the facial nerve should be tested in all its divisions. The parotid and submandibular ducts should be inspected to assess saliva flow, redness and the presence of pus or an obvious stone. The mouth should be inspected to see if it is excessively dry.

After inspection, the glands should be palpated carefully by bimanual exploration. It is only in this way that a proper assessment can be made. The ducts should be felt carefully for calculi and then massaged gently towards the opening to express any pus present.

The patient can be given an acid-drop to suck and any enlargement on salivation assessed.

The ears should be inspected to make sure that there is no salivary fistula or tumour extension through the anterior meatal wall.

Gentle probing of the duct may produce a gush of turbid saliva.

INVESTIGATION

1 Plain X-ray, including occlusal views, will show a radio-opaque calculus.

2 Ultrasonic scanning of the gland is quick, non-invasive and exposes the patient to no radiation. It will identify masses, cysts and calculi but is only comprehensible to the radiologist!

3 Sialography will outline the duct system. Contrast medium is injected into the gland after cannulation of the duct, and will show radiolucent stones or strictures. A solid tumour will not fill with contrast, but an area of sialectasis will be seen as droplets in the dilated ducts. Sialography contributes little to tumour diagnosis and is not usually performed in such cases.

4 If there is a large parotid tumour with parapharyngeal extension, an MR scan will outline its extent.

Acute inflammation

Mumps

Mumps is the commonest acute inflammatory condition of salivary glands. It affects mainly the parotid glands, which become uniformly swollen and painful, but the submandibular glands may also be involved. Its incidence had fallen to very low levels as a result of immunization, but is now rising alarmingly as some parents decline to have their children immunized.

Acute suppurative parotitis

Acute suppurative parotitis is uncommon and usually occurs in debilitated patients. Treatment is with antibiotics, rehydration and oral hygiene. If an abscess develops, surgical incision is required.

Acute sialadenitis

Acute sialadenitis may affect the submandibular gland (commonly) or the parotid gland (rarely) because of the presence of a duct calculus. The affected gland is painful and swollen and is made worse by eating. The patient is usually unwell with a pyrexia.

Removal of the stone provides dramatic relief in most cases.

Recurrent acute inflammation

Recurrent acute inflammation of the major salivary glands presents a problem of management if no stone is present. If there is a duct stricture, gentle dilatation may be curative. In childhood, recurrent episodes of acute inflammation will usually subside by puberty and should be treated conservatively.

Chronic inflammation

Chronic inflammation of the parotid or submandibular gland is usually due to sialectasis (duct dilatation leading to stasis and infection) and will not usually respond to conservative measures. The gland is thickened with episodic pain and infection, and can be felt easily on bimanual examination.

TREATMENT

The submandibular gland so affected can be excised; chronic sialectasis of the parotid poses a difficult problem. Excision has a high risk of facial nerve damage and long-term antibiotics should be tried before resorting to parotidectomy.

Sjögren's syndrome

Sjögren's syndrome is an auto-immune systemic disorder affecting the salivary and lacrimal glands. There is enlargement of the glands and loss of secretion, leading to dryness of the eyes and mouth. In many cases, biopsy of the lip mucosa will show minor salivary glands heavily infiltrated by lymphocytes. Symptomatic relief can be obtained by the use of artificial saliva or glycerin and warm-water mouthwash.

Salivary retention cysts

Salivary cysts occur most commonly in the floor of the mouth, where they may become very large and expand the loose tissues (Fig. 40.2). The name 'ranula' is often applied. Less commonly, such retention cysts occur on the mucosal aspect of the lips.

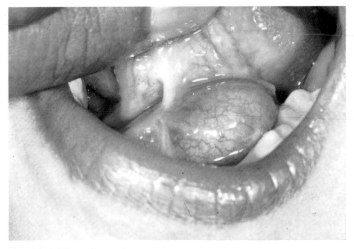

Fig. 40.2 Sublingual retention cyst.

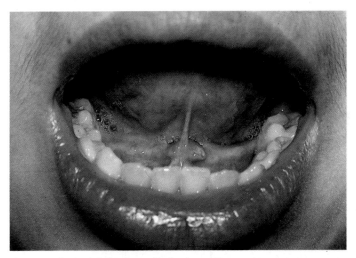

Fig. 40.3 Calculus in left submandibular duct orifice.

Salivary calculi

Most salivary calculi occur in the submandibular gland because of the mucoid nature of its saliva, which can become inspissated (Fig. 40.3). However, calculi do also occur in the parotid gland.

CLINICAL FEATURES

The flow of saliva from the affected gland becomes obstructed, causing the gland to swell during salivation. Such swelling is painful and its size may be alarming. The swelling will usually resolve over about an hour.

The calculus can be seen if it presents at the duct opening, or felt within the duct or gland.

INVESTIGATION

Most, but not all, calculi are radio-opaque, and X-rays should be performed as described above.

TREATMENT

1   Intraductal calculi can be removed from the duct under local anaesthetic. A suture should first be passed around the duct proximal to the stone to prevent its movement back into the gland. Removal of such a stone may be more difficult than you might expect.

2   If the stone is within the substance of the salivary gland, excision of the gland will have to be considered. The submandibular gland presents no problem as it is straightforward to excise, but parotidectomy for calculus requires a high degree of skill.

Salivary gland tumours

Salivary glands, because they contain lymph nodes within their structure, may be the site of metastases from a non-salivary primary site or from blood dyscrasias such as leukaemia (Fig. 40.4). Salivary gland disease is uncommon in childhood, but a solid parotid tumour presenting under the age of 16 is more likely (60:40) than not to be malignant.

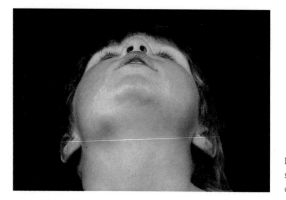

Fig. 40.4 Enlarged right submandibular gland from chronic infection.

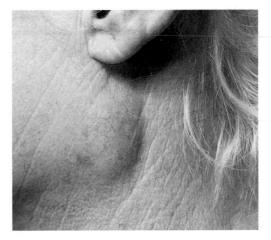

Fig. 40.5 A pleomorphic adenoma in the tail of the parotid gland.

It is not usually possible to detect clinically whether a tumour in a salivary gland is benign or malignant. Fine needle aspiration cytology may be helpful in predicting the type of tumour present. All such tumours should be treated as malignant until the diagnosis is confirmed by histology. The same tumours occur in minor salivary glands as in the major glands but malignant tumours in minor glands have a more aggressive course.

PATHOLOGICAL CLASSIFICATION

Benign tumours

Pleomorphic salivary adenoma (mixed salivary tumour, PSA)
(Fig. 40.5)
Occurs most frequently in the parotid gland. Propensity for recurrence if not removed with surrounding cuff of tissue. PSA accounts for about 90% of parotid tumours in adults.

Warthin's tumour (cystic lymphoepithelial lesion)
Almost exclusive to the parotid gland, it causes a smooth swelling in the tail of the gland that may feel cystic.

Haemangioma
A rare tumour, usually congenital or occurring in early childhood; occurs most commonly in the parotid gland. A haemangioma is also often present on the skin of the face or in the mouth.

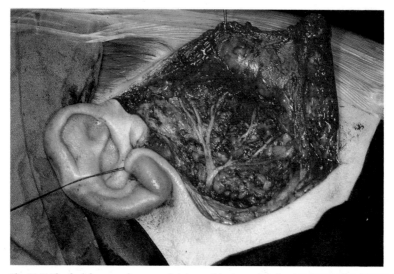

Fig. 40.6 The facial nerve after superficial parotidectomy for a benign tumour in a boy aged 12 years.

Malignant tumours

Adenoid cystic carcinoma

The commonest malignant tumour of salivary glands. With early perineural invasion, the long-term prognosis is poor but survival for many years is usual.

Muco-epidermoid tumours

Can arise in any of the salivary glands and have a variable degree of malignancy; the majority will behave as benign tumours but a small proportion are aggressively malignant.

Acinic cell tumours

Are usually of low-grade malignancy and occur almost exclusively in the parotid gland.

Malignant pleomorphic adenomata

May arise in an existing adenoma. The malignant change is made apparent by a rapid increase in size and, in the case of parotid tumours, the development of facial weakness. A benign tumour causes no such weakness.

Squamous carcinoma

Squamous carcinoma of the submandibular and parotid glands is uncommon and has a very poor prognosis. Radical excision followed by radiotherapy is the only treatment that offers any chance of cure.

Lymphoma

Lymphoma can occur in any of the salivary glands, major or minor. Surgery has no part in treatment other than for biopsy, but radiotherapy and/or chemotherapy may be curative. The lymphoma arises from lymphoid tissue within the salivary gland.

Salivary incontinence (drooling)

While not due to disease of the salivary glands, children or adults with, for example, cerebral palsy or stroke may be unable to control the saliva produced, particularly from the sublingual and submandibular ducts. This results in much distress and discomfort to patient and relatives. It can often be relieved by surgical relocation of the submandibular ducts to a posterior position near the tonsil combined with excision of the sublingual gland.

Surgery of the salivary glands

SUBMANDIBULAR GLAND EXCISION

This is usually performed for tumour removal but may be made necessary by calculus or by chronic infection. The gland is approached externally and care is taken not to damage the marginal mandibular branch of the facial nerve or the lingual nerve.

PAROTIDECTOMY

Again, usually undertaken for removal of tumour (Fig. 40.6). The facial nerve is identified at an early stage in the operation and its branches followed carefully. Usually the tumour lies superficial to the nerve but if it is deep, the nerve will need to be mobilized. All patients having parotidectomy must be warned of the risk of facial nerve damage.

Index

Page references in *italics* refer to figures